T0212829

SpringerBriefs in Public Health

Series Editor
Angelo P. Giardino
Houston
Texas
USA

SpringerBriefs in Public Health present concise summaries of cutting-edge research and practical applications from across the entire field of public health, with contributions from medicine, bioethics, health economics, public policy, biostatistics, and sociology.

The focus of the series is to highlight current topics in public health of interest to a global audience, including health care policy; social determinants of health; health issues in developing countries; new research methods; chronic and infectious disease epidemics; and innovative health interventions.

Featuring compact volumes of 50–125 pages, the series covers a range of content from professional to academic. Possible volumes in the series may consist of timely reports of state-of-the art analytical techniques, reports from the field, snapshots of hot and/or emerging topics, elaborated theses, literature reviews, and in-depth case studies. Both solicited and unsolicited manuscripts are considered for publication in this series.

Briefs are published as part of Springer's eBook collection, with millions of users worldwide. In addition, Briefs are available for individual print and electronic purchase.

Briefs are characterized by fast, global electronic dissemination, standard publishing contracts, easy-to-use manuscript preparation and formatting guidelines, and expedited production schedules. We aim for publication 8–12 weeks after acceptance.

More information about this series at http://www.springer.com/series/10138

David D. Schwartz • Marni E. Axelrad

Healthcare Partnerships for Pediatric Adherence

Promoting Collaborative Management for Pediatric Chronic Illness Care

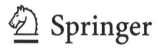 Springer

David D. Schwartz
Associate Professor of Pediatrics
Department of Pediatrics
Section of Psychology
Baylor College of Medicine
Houston
Texas
USA

Marni E. Axelrad
Associate Professor of Pediatrics
Department of Pediatrics
Section of Psychology
Baylor College of Medicine
Houston
Texas
USA

ISSN 2192-3698   ISSN 2192-3701 (electronic)
SpringerBriefs in Public Health
ISBN 978-3-319-13667-7   ISBN 978-3-319-13668-4 (eBook)
DOI 10.1007/978-3-319-13668-4

Library of Congress Control Number: 2015935622

Springer Cham Heidelberg New York Dordrecht London

Printed on acid-free paper

Springer is part of Springer Science+Business Media (www.springer.com)

Preface

Advances in treatment and management of pediatric chronic illness have resulted in substantial improvements in the health of children and youth. But, to paraphrase former U.S. Surgeon General C. Everett Koop, treatments don't work in patients who don't follow them.

Nonadherence—not following a treatment regimen as prescribed—is believed to be the single greatest cause of treatment failure, resulting in significant morbidity and mortality, and costing hundreds of billions of dollars per year. It is also one of the most challenging and frustrating problems facing clinicians, who often do not know not how to help their patients struggling with adherence. Over the past 20 years, there have been significant advances in our understanding of nonadherence and in the development of empirically-supported interventions, yet there has been virtually no change in overall rates of nonadherence. The reasons for this discrepancy between research findings and population health form the core of this book, which is intended to help bridge the gap between research advances and lagging improvements in children's health. This volume provides a comprehensive educational resource for physicians, nurses, psychologists, social workers an any other healthcare professionals who work with children and adolescents and their families and try to help them with the often overwhelming task of managing a chronic illness.

In this volume we argue that progress in reducing nonadherence has been limited by intervention efforts that have been fragmented and poorly integrated, targeting one or at best a few of the factors known to affect adherence, to the relative neglect of others. For example, interventions may target patient motivation without addressing contributing family factors or barriers to access to care. While this approach is sensible in the research setting, it neglects the co-morbidities and complications that characterize most patients who present with adherence difficulties in "real world" clinical settings. Managing these complexities requires a systematic approach that addresses all the major contributing factors to nonadherence in a comprehensive, integrated fashion. The overarching theme is that successful illness management depends on developing "healthcare partnerships" between patients, families, and healthcare providers, and on providing support for families to navigate the complex healthcare system.

This volume includes practical guidelines for clinicians to screen for nonadherence; a model for patient triage to different levels and types of intervention; best practices for interventions for different problems; suggestions for fostering family teamwork; and education for professionals on how best to promote and support health-maintaining behaviors in their patients. As such it should be of value to all clinicians who wish to help children and their families be more successful with illness management. The book also provides a rough blueprint for developing an integrated system for promoting good adherence and preventing or reducing nonadherence that that should be of significant interest to clinical directors, administrators, and policy-makers.

In Part I, we provide a broad but detailed overview of the topic of pediatric adherence. **Chapter 1** provides the background into the concept of adherence and the scope and impact of nonadherence. It also discusses some barriers to adherence inherent in the healthcare system as it is currently constituted, and introduces the partnership model. **Chapter 2** selectively reviews important theoretical models of adherence and relevant constructs, laying these out from initial adaptation through the different processes that underlie patient adherence. **Chapter 3** provides an up-to-date review of the research literature on barriers and facilitators of adherence, and **Chap. 4** reviews the research on effective interventions for nonadherence. In Chaps. 5 and 6 we discussed developmental issues as they pertain to illness management. **Chapter 5** discusses management in early to middle childhood, while **Chap. 6** focuses on adolescence, the period when adherence is at its worst. In the latter chapter we review recent research from developmental neurobiology and focus on risk taking, and argue that poor adherence in adolescence is likely to be the norm, as a result of normal aspects of adolescent development. In **Chap. 7** we discuss the critical role parents play in helping their children manage a chronic illness. In the next two chapters, we focus on some of the most vulnerable patients with chronic illness. **Chapter 8** focuses on families struggling with poverty. Poverty creates significant challenges to managing a child's chronic illness, leading many authors and clinicians to despair of finding effective solutions to help these vulnerable families; however, we believe that progress can be made by focusing on reducing chronic stress and fostering the buffering relationships within families. **Chapter 9** discusses health disparities in adherence for racial/ethnic minorities, and focuses on provider-family communication as both a contributor to problematic adherence and as an important variable to target for intervention.

In Part II, we present a conceptual model of collaborative care around pediatric adherence. In **Chap. 10**, we begin by arguing for a reconsideration of the idea of self-management, and join other authors in support of a more collaborative, family centered approach. The idea of a triadic partnership between patients, parents, and their healthcare providers is discussed in **Chap. 11**, with many practical suggestions for how pediatricians and other providers can foster such partnerships with their patients.

Finally, in Part III, we present a comprehensive, integrated model for improving the care we provide to children with chronic illness and their families in promoting better adherence. **Chapter 12** discusses methods for screening for nonadherence and contributory psychosocial problems in children with chronic illness, and in **Chap. 13** we present a model program for providing comprehensive assessment and intervention services based on level and type of assessed risk/need. The model cuts across different modalities, addressing patient, family, and provider factors in an integrated fashion. **Chap. 14** provides a brief summary of the main clinical implications of the literature reviewed in this volume.

A Few Notes

Acute versus chronic illness. Adherence issues affect both acute and chronic healthcare management. Adherence to medications for acute illnesses such as infections is an important health issue, especially at the population level, but the focus of this book will be primarily on adherence in chronic conditions. Nonadherence is generally higher in chronic conditions and is associated with greater patient morbidity. More importantly from the perspective of this volume, managing a chronic condition is qualitatively different from managing an acute illness. Acute illnesses by definition are time-limited, and place different demands upon families and family resources. As discussed later on, chronic illness becomes a chronic *stressor* which requires continual readjustments from patient and family, and unfortunately management burnout is common, contributing to a host of complicating factors including parent-child conflict and depression.

  A note on the word "parent." Throughout this volume we use the term "parent" to refer to the child's primary caregiver or caregivers. We recognize that many children are actually being raised by other adults, whether they be grandparents or other relatives, foster parents, or others *in loco parentis,* and we do not mean to diminish the importance of these individuals. In fact, we wish to highlight their importance by using the term *parent* to refer to anyone in the parenting role—i.e., in the role of caring for the child. In our experience, these other persons are often thought of as parents by the child in their care, and think of themselves in this light as well. We have opted against using the more generic term *caregiver* as we believe that it places too much emphasis on the functional role and too little on the emotional role that comes with parenting.

Acknowledgements

We would like to thank Doug Ris for his support and encouragement while writing this volume, and Cortney Taylor for her help with some of the background research. Most importantly, this volume would not have been possible without the guiding influence of Barbara Anderson, who has always stressed the critical importance of family and family teamwork in chronic illness care. We are very appreciative of all of the children and families who have participated in our research. And finally, we thank our own children, who waited so patiently for us to finish.

Contents

Part I
Snapshot from the Field

Current Practice and Policy

Chapter 1
Introduction: Definitions, Scope, and Impact of Nonadherence

Abstract Nonadherence is believed to be the single greatest cause of treatment failure, resulting in substantial morbidity and mortality, much of which could have been avoided. In this chapter we review the scope of the problem of nonadherence, and discuss definitional issues including the distinctions between disease and illness; compliance, adherence, and nonadherence; and intentional and unintentional nonadherence. The multi-factorial nature of nonadherence is highlighted. Barriers inherent in the current healthcare system are then reviewed with an eye toward identifying areas where more improvement could be made.

Introduction

> From the patient's perspective, the question is not why patients choose to be less than fully adherent, but, rather, why they choose to take any treatment to begin with.—Adams et al. 2004

The prevalence of pediatric chronic conditions severe enough to cause disability has increased dramatically over the past 20 years, with recent prevalence rates suggesting that as many as half of all children may have a chronic condition at some point in time (Cleave et al. 2010). Illnesses such as diabetes, end-stage organ disease, and asthma cause substantial suffering, and can require burdensome daily management—such as taking medication or making significant changes in diet—that can greatly reduce a child's quality of life. Even when some conditions are "cured," such as when a child with organ failure receives a transplant, daily medical treatments often must continue to ensure the child remains healthy.

As noted in the Preface, nonadherence is thought to be the single greatest cause of treatment failure, resulting in preventable complications of illness that at their most severe can include organ failure, brain damage, and premature death (e.g., Dobbels et al. 2010; Oliva et al. 2013; Simoni et al. 2007; Wolfsdorf et al. 2009). It has therefore been suggested that "increasing the effectiveness of adherence interventions may have a far greater impact on the health of the population than any improvement

© Springer International Publishing Switzerland 2015
D. D. Schwartz, M. E. Axelrad, *Healthcare Partnerships for Pediatric Adherence,*
SpringerBriefs in Public Health, DOI 10.1007/978-3-319-13668-4_1

in specific medical treatments" (Haynes 2001). Nonadherence can also complicate clinical decision-making, resulting in unnecessary changes in medication or dosage, and it is a major cause of emergency room visits and hospital admissions, resulting in excess care costing hundreds of billions of dollars in the U.S. each year (DiMatteo 2004). For over 20 years, we have known that approximately half of all medical treatments are not followed as prescribed (e.g., Rapoff and Barnard 1991), and these rates have effectively remained unchanged (see Stark 2013) despite the development of interventions shown to be effective at reducing nonadherent behaviors across a range of pediatric medical conditions (Kahana et al. 2008), resulting in significant improvements in children's health (Graves et al. 2010).

Why have we made no real dent in the overall problem of pediatric nonadherence despite making substantial progress in development of effective interventions? It is well understood that nonadherence is a multi-factorial problem involving multiple actors and systems, including the patient, the family, the healthcare team, the broader healthcare system, society and culture (Rapoff 2010; Sabaté 2003), yet clinical and research efforts have tended to focus on one or a few components to the relative neglect of the others. Substantial changes in rates of nonadherence will likely not occur unless efforts to promote adherence become less fragmented and address all the major components in a systematic fashion, which is the conclusion reached by the World Health Organization over a decade ago (Sabete 2003). The challenge is in designing a system that can be implemented in the current healthcare environment.

Managing a chronic illness is complicated; and as treatments have improved, the level of regimen complexity has only increased (Hood et al. 2009). Types of adherence behavior include: taking medication, either in pill or liquid form, through subcutaneous injections, an inhaler, or other means (e.g., insulin pump); changes to diet and/or fluid intake; and other lifestyle modifications such as exercise. Individuals often have to complete multiple illness management behaviors, monitor and keep track of what they have done (e.g., tracking taking a daily pill, keeping a glucose log book), and adapt their daily schedule to accommodate management. Some conditions require reviewing health data (e.g., pattern management in diabetes), and making adjustments to the regimen either with or without direct guidance from the physician.

Appointment-keeping is another adherence behavior that does not always receive the same attention as regimen adherence (Schwartz et al. 2010). Patients with chronic illness who do not see their healthcare providers at recommended intervals tend to have worse health than those who do (Kaufman et al. 1999). This is the "Catch-22" in helping patients who struggle with adherence, as these patients also tend to have lower service utilization, whether it involves keeping medical appointments, or utilizing behavioral health supports that can make adherence more manageable (Schwartz et al. 2011). Of course, in pediatrics, clinic attendance is largely or completely a *parental* adherence behavior, even into later adolescence. This highlights another important theme of this book; namely, that pediatric illness management has to be considered in the context of *family adherence*.

"Illness" versus "Disease"

If you ask patients and their healthcare providers the purpose of medical treatment—and medical adherence—you might receive very different answers. In general, healthcare professionals are focusing on controlling disease course and progression, helping a patient maintain physical homeostasis (e.g., blood sugars, blood pressure), and limiting complications. For patients, treatments are primarily about controlling symptoms and *feeling better right now*, and often only secondarily about reducing complications.

These different views of treatment align with differences in the conception of what it means to be sick. Patients and their providers often view the phenomenon of being sick from very different angles. The healthcare profession, of course, is trained in the medical model, which views disease as an objectively measurable condition due to some pathogenic entity or process that disrupts normal bodily function. A disease in this sense is the same regardless of who has it. Patients and their families, on the other hand, view being sick as a *state of being* that afflicts the person, often causing pain or discomfort, sometimes limiting daily activities, and frequently carrying social stigma. Importantly, the same underlying pathogenic factor can be experienced very differently be different people. Being sick may often also have very different meanings for different people. *Explanatory models* of sickness are strongly influenced by culture. Many traditional societies view being sick as a manifestation of supernatural forces; many people continue to view being ill as a manifestation of personal weakness, or as punishment for wrong-doing.

In a classic paper, Cassell (1976) suggested that the term *illness* be used to capture a person's subjective experience and understanding (what it *means* to the person to be sick), whereas *disease* should refer to the physical-medical entity familiar to doctors and other healthcare professionals. Or, in his own words,

> Let us use the word 'illness' to stand for what the patient feels when he goes to the doctor and 'disease' for what he has on the way home from the doctor's office. Disease, then is something an organ has; illness is something a man has.

As suggested by Helman (1981), "most cases of disease, though not all, are accompanied by illness," and many cases of illness, but not all, will reflect an underlying disease. However, as the focus of this volume is on management of pediatric chronic diseases such as diabetes or asthma, we will not be covering the case of illness without disease.

An important corollary of the disease/illness distinction is that, generally speaking, patients and their families focus on treating *illness* whereas doctors focus on treating *disease*. As a result, their treatment goals may differ significantly, although it is often the case that neither party is aware of this difference. Nonadherence often reflects this difference in viewpoint. For example, children are less adherent to asthma medication when they are asymptomatic (van Es et al. 1998) even discontinuing medication use when symptoms are well controlled and they feel well, because they see no further need for treatment (Bender et al. 2000). At the same time, physicians frequently communicate solely in biomedical terms (Roter et al. 1997), which is associated with lower patient satisfaction (Ashton et al. 2003), rather than asking patients about their experiences and beliefs, which has been noted to improve the patient-provider relationship (Street et al. 2008). An important contention of this volume is that a lack of concordance between a patient's (and family's) illness-centered viewpoint and healthcare provider's disease-centered viewpoint leads to communication breakdowns that can significantly affect adherence.

Definition of Adherence and Nonadherence

Adherence has been defined as "the extent to which a person's behavior—taking medication, following diet, or executing lifestyle changes—corresponds with agreed recommendations from a health care provider" (Sabate 2003). Adherence means more than just following physician instructions. Patients and their families take an active role in adopting and maintaining health management behaviors over time, and this can require significant changes for the whole family. Current treatment regimens can be quite complex and demanding, may involve significant disruption of children's daily lives, and over time frequently results in burnout for youth and increased levels of conflict in families. The often overwhelming burden of daily adherence cannot be overstated. Modi et al. (2012) also make the interesting point that "adherence is socially constructed and would not exist without an interchange between patients and providers" (e475). As will be seen, the reality is that patient-provider agreement is often more aspirational than actual, and patients and providers often have different views on their degree of concordance; but at least the intent of using the term *adherence* is to give more prominence to patient input in illness management decisions.

The term *compliance* has traditionally been used to refer to whether or not patients followed medical advice. The term has been losing favor as the field of medicine moves away from provider-centric models of care towards patient-centered care (Epstein and Street 2011), the idea being that *compliance* means doing what the provider says, whereas *adherence* carries a stronger connotation of agreement between patient and healthcare providers. However, both terms remain in current use.

Another term starting to be used in the literature is *self-management* (Glasgow 2008; Lorig and Holman 2003; Modi et al. 2012). Glasgow (2008) suggested that "the term self-management is preferred over adherence or compliance to reflect the role of agency and self-determination involved in health-promoting or disease management behaviors." Modi et al. (2012) argued that self-management is a broader term than adherence, encompassing adherence to health behaviors, contextual factors (individual, family, health care system, community influences) that impact the execution of those behaviors, and self-management processes such as decision-making. In this model the term *adherence* attains greater specificity, allowing for more precise operationalization of the frequency of specific treatment behaviors.

More recently, the term *concordance* has also been used, especially in the UK. Concordance typically implies a very active, shared decision-making process between patients, families, and their healthcare providers (Horne et al. 2005). As noted by Santer et al. (2014), this sort of shared decision-making is more aspirational than actual in common practice. In fact, taking such an active role is difficult for families as well as providers (Adams et al. 2004), and we currently have a very limited understanding of how to best make this sort of shared decision-making work.

Scope of the Problem of Nonadherence

Problematic Adherence is the Primary Cause of Treatment Failure Unfortunately, poor adherence is quite common among children and (especially) adolescents. It is estimated that approximately 20–30% of medication prescriptions are never filled (Viswanathan et al. 2012), and 50–55% of pediatric patients do not consistently adhere to medical regimens for chronic conditions (Rapoff 2010). This figure does not mean that 50% of *children* are nonadherent, but that 50% of *treatments* are not completed as prescribed. Thus, the scope of problematic adherence is likely even greater, in terms of the number of people involved. For example, one large study of diabetes centers in Europe found that *over 90%* of youth reported intentionally omitting insulin at least once per month. While this may sound relatively minor, missing insulin can cause a diabetic child to experience diabetic ketoacidosis (DKA), a life-threatening metabolic crisis that can cause coma, permanent brain damage, and death. Nonadherence to insulin is the primary cause of DKA in children with established diabetes (Wolfsdorf et al. 2009). Similarly, incomplete adherence to immunosuppressive drugs is known to be the primary cause of heart, kidney, and liver transplant failures in adolescents (Dobbels et al. 2010; Oliva et al. 2013; Shemesh 2004), and it is a leading cause of treatment failure in children infected with human immunodeficiency virus (HIV) (Simoni et al. 2007).

Suboptimal adherence has other costs as well. Recent estimates suggest that nonadherence results in monetary losses of hundreds of billion dollars annually in the U.S. alone (Viswanathan et al. 2012). The financial impact is especially trenchant in an era when healthcare costs are soaring and society is struggling to continue to afford first-class care. Much of this cost derives from expensive emergency room visits and hospital admissions (Laffel et al. 1998; Maldonado et al. 2003; Svoren et al. 2003) that result from avoidable exacerbations of illness, which place additional strain on an already over-taxed healthcare system. Nonadherence can also complicate clinical decision-making, resulting in unnecessary changes in medication or dosage (DiMatteo 2004), and research into the efficacy of medications can be affected by variability in participants' adherence to the study drug or other intervention (Rapoff 2010).

The focus of this book is on pediatric adherence in the United States. However, it should be acknowledged that poor treatment adherence for chronic diseases is actually "a worldwide problem of striking magnitude" according to the World Health Organization (Sabate 2003). Adherence rates are even lower in developing countries, where the disease burden is even higher, and healthcare systems are even more pressed to provide basic services.

Adherence is Not An All-or-none Phenomenon In trying to understand adherence (and nonadherence), it is important to recognize that adherence is not an all-or-none, either-or phenomenon. It is probably true that *all* people are "nonadherent" at some point in time, to a greater or lesser degree. The reader can probably think of times when he or she did not finish a course of antibiotics, or skipped flossing after a meal, or deviated from a diet. The daily management requirements faced by individuals with chronic illness only make nonadherence more likely, by creating more opportunities to not complete some management task.

Adherence can vary by behavior (a patient does X but not Y), frequency (a patient completes only X % of treatment), and time. Children may adhere consistently to one part of their healthcare regimen while completing a second management behavior intermittently and fully neglecting a third. A child with type 1 diabetes might never miss an insulin dose, but only check blood glucose levels once or twice a day; or she might take long-acting insulin regularly but avoid taking her short-acting insulin; or she might take all insulin and check blood sugars regularly but "guestimate" how many carbs she has eaten rather than complete a full calculation. In fact, it has generally been found that adherence to one management behavior does not necessarily predict adherence to others. Comparing across behaviors, adherence to medication is generally highest, with lifestyle changes (i.e., changes in diet and exercise) being most problematic (Rapoff 2010).

Adherence behaviors also vary over time. Adherence after diagnosis is typically high, declining to some degree over time as management fatigue sets in. It is not uncommon for a youth with excellent illness management to "burn out" and suddenly show a significant drop-off in self-care. Youth have also been know to take brief "drug holidays" (for example, when going on an overnight with friends), which can result in symptom exacerbations and worse. The end of the school year also entails some risk of a decline in adherence, as the structure and schedule of school (and availability of a school nurse) give way to the vagaries of summer. It is also clear that adherence changes during certain developmental periods, adolescence in particular (see Chap. 6). It is not always easy to predict who might show a change in adherence behavior over time, although identifying risk factors for a decline in adherence is an active area of research (Schwartz et al. 2013; see Chap. 12).

Recognizing that adherence varies by behavior and over time leads to the realization that there really is no such thing as "a nonadherent patient." Nonadherence is not a quality of a person, but the outcome of a specific behavior at a particular point in time, in interaction with multiple contextual factors (Modi et al. 2012). Healthcare providers often suggest that some patients are more "difficult" than others, and while there may be some subjective truth in this, the factors that contribute to this difficulty are complex and often result from *interactions* between the patient, his family, his healthcare providers, and/or the healthcare system—which is a core theme of this book. In other words, so-called difficult patients may only be difficult under certain circumstances.

Focusing on specific adherence behaviors rather than on a presumed characteristic of a patient also has pragmatic benefits—adherence behaviors are concrete, measurable, and amenable to change (La Greca and Bearman 2001). Moreover, clinical experience suggests that patients are much more likely to be receptive to (and successful at) working on changing a specific behavior or behaviors than working on changing "who they are."

> Perhaps it is time to give "adherence" a rest and instead focus on the "treatment-related behaviors" we try to promote in children and families. One benefit of shifting our thinking and conceptualization is that it might also reduce the negative and paternalistic connotations associated with "adherence." (La Greca and Bearman 2001)

Viewing illness management from the standpoint of specific adherence behaviors also helps resolve a longstanding conundrum: how to operationalize nonadherence. Is a patient who takes less than 80% of his medication nonadherent, as convention would have it (Rapoff 2010)? What about the patient who takes 90% of her medication but only follows dietary restrictions half the time? Obviously, "optimal" rates will have to be defined by illness (e.g., higher adherence for HIV treatments; Chesney 2003), adherence behavior (e.g., a diabetes patient missing glucose checks versus missing insulin doses), and in the clinical realm, for each individual patient. Adams et al. (2004) suggest using an adherence index by dividing the amount of medication taken by the amount prescribed.

A huge advantage of this sort of calculation is that it adds needed precision both to clinical care and to research (Modi et al. 2012). It also moves families and physicians away from subjective judgments of "good" and "bad" adherence (Wolpert and Anderson 2001), and allows them to set small, attainable goals (for example, increasing glucose checks from 1x/day to 2x/day) that can then be built on. As noted by Wolpert and Anderson, "goals that are too ambitious and overlook the realities of the patient's life can be a set up for failure," whereas setting attainable goals, "even if they are far from ideal, will foster a sense of success, competence, and engagement that can drive greater improvements as the goals are further advanced."

The observations above raise the difficult question of measurement of adherence. For example, should a practitioner rely on parent report or child self-report of adherence, neither of which is very reliable? More objective assessments (e.g., pill counters, prescription refill rates) are more reliable but also costly and probably not feasible for regular use in clinical contexts. Perhaps a good compromise is for clinicians to use standardized rating scales, a number of which have well established reliability and validity and are easy to use (see Quittner et al. 2008 for review). While these measures are valuable, practitioners should be cautious about using combined measures that provide an overall index of adherence. Consider again the finding that 90% of youth with type 1 diabetes disclosed intentional insulin omission; presumably a significant proportion of those youth would score below cut-off for nonadherence on an overall measure of nonadherence, so that the risky behavior (omitting insulin) would be missed. It might be important for providers to use a general (screening) assessment of adherence for all patients, as well as following up about more specific management behaviors (Modi et al. 2012) for those patients having difficulty with illness control.

Given the above, we question the clinical and empirical value of the term "non-adherence." In almost all cases, patients are not "not adherent," they are almost always partially adherent, with differing rates of adherence to different behaviors at different times. Reframing the problem of nonadherence as one of difficulty maintaining consistent adherence to certain, specific behaviors is not only more accurate but it also avoids the negative connotations of "not" doing something, which implies a refusal to engage in the behavior. In our experience, referring to a patient as nonadherent is all too often associated with seeing the patient as difficult, as not doing what she is told—which is exactly what the field of medicine has tried to avoid by more or less abandoning the term *noncompliance*, which was seen (correctly) as too provider-oriented and authoritarian, and not patient-centered and collaborative. When we use the term *nonadherence* in this book, it will be used in the very specific sense of not engaging in the behavior in question—what has in other work been termed *intentional nonadherence* (Adams et al. 2004).

Intentional and Unintentional Adherence   *Unintentional* (or *inadvertent*) *nonadherence* reflects factors typically out of the patient's control, such as lack of insurance coverage for prescribed care, or forgetting to take medicine. Forgetting is often the most common reason given by patients for missing treatments (Anderson 2012; Buchanan et al. 2012; Penza-Clyve et al. 2004) although it is possible that forgetting may simply be the most socially acceptable response (Adams et al. 2004). Unintentional nonadherence may be more likely among families with lower SES (Wroe 2002), probably because resource limitations complicate the organizational demands of illness management.

In contrast, *intentional* (or *volitional*) *nonadherence* refers to the fact that adherence behaviors reflect choices made by the patient or parent (Adams et al. 2004; Wroe 2002). Patients may decide to omit or reduce the frequency of an adherence behavior or change dose to manage side-effects, or because of perceived detriments that outweigh benefits (e.g., deciding against stimulant medication for ADHD due to parent fears of addiction; Charach et al. 2014), or to avoid stigma (e.g., a youth with diabetes who refuses to check blood glucose or take insulin in front of friends). As Adams et al. (2004) note, "little is known about the fundamental process of decision-making as it pertains to volitional nonadherence," although in Chap. 6 we provide some speculations based on recent research on adolescent decision-making.

Adams et al. (2004) make the important point that many interventions focus on inadvertent or unintentional nonadherence (e.g., use of reminders and cues), an approach that is not likely to be successful for nonadherence that is volitional. Understanding the *type* of nonadherent behavior is crucial to being able to intervene effectively. They also note that intentional and unintentional behaviors lie on a continuum. This is an important point. For example, in adults, there is evidence that "unintentional" nonadherence is predicted by patients' health beliefs (Gadkari and McHorney 2012), suggesting it may not be purely accidental.

Perhaps a better way to understand nonadherence that is neither intentional nor accidental is through the concept of *behavioral willingness* (Gibbons and Gerrard 1997), which has been defined as "an openness to risk opportunity—what an individual would be willing to do under some circumstances" (Gibbons 2008). In this formulation, most risk behavior is a predisposed "reaction to social circumstances" rather than intentional, although one might argue that there *is* an intent, it is just arrived at on the spur-of-the-moment, reflecting a quick decision rather than being the result of a more deliberative process. In this context, nonadherence would be conceptualized as a behavior that results from a last minute decision—for example, a diabetic adolescent who runs out with friends and decides against running back in for his glucometer. These sorts of decisions have been called "nonintentional but volitional" risk behaviors (Gerrard et al. 2008), and we would argue that they fall somewhere between intentional and unintentional behaviors, as they reflect true decisions that are unplanned.

Is Nonadherence Intractable? The huge scope of the problem of nonadherence is not news. Over 10 years ago, the World Health Organization put out a comprehensive report on the phenomenon of nonadherence worldwide, calling poor treatment adherence "a worldwide problem of striking magnitude" (Sabate 2003). More recently, the Agency for Healthcare Research and Quality published a similar report of findings, with similar results and similar conclusions (Viswanathan et al. 2012). Tellingly, there has been no change in the estimated prevalence of nonadherence over the years, which seems to be stuck at about 50%, a figure that dates at least to 1979 (Haynes et al. 1979) and continues to be cited with regularity (see Rapoff 2010 for a recent review of prevalence estimates across different pediatric conditions). Brown and Bussel (2011) go so far as to suggest that the problem of poor adherence goes all the way back to the time of Hippocrates, over 2000 years ago! Moreover, the 50% rule-of-thumb is applicable both to adults as well as children, a continuity with serious implications for pediatric adherence, especially in adolescence when youth are typically given primary responsibility for managing their illness. For if adults struggle so much with adherence, how can we expect children to do better?

The good news is there *are* effective psychosocial interventions for promoting and improving adherence (Chap. 4). In general, the most effective interventions are behavioral, or include a behavioral component, and are implemented or developed/supervised by psychologists. Effect sizes are relatively modest but often clinically significant. For example, a meta-analysis of adherence interventions for children and youth with type 1 diabetes (Winkley et al. 2006) reported a mean effect size of psychological intervention on glycemic control of -0.035, which they explain translates into a pooled reduction in hemoglobin A1c of 0.5%. While this might not sound like a lot, a reduction of this magnitude lowers relative risk for microvascular complications by about 15%, heart attack by 5–10%, and diabetes-related death by about 10%. Effect sizes for pulmonary function in asthma were even larger ($d = 1.01$; Graves et al. 2010). Moreover, small effects can result in substantial improvements in health when spread across a population. Why, then, has there been no evident change in overall prevalence of nonadherence?

One reason, which we return to in Chap. 12, is that adherence problems are often identified too late, after they have become set patterns that are difficult to change. A second factor is the multi-dimensional nature of adherence—without an integrated, multi-level approach to intervention, important factors that contribute to nonadherence are likely to be missed (Chap. 13). There are also systemic reasons why nonadherence remains such a resistant problem, as we discuss in the next section.

The Current Healthcare System is Not Set Up to Promote Adherence to Chronic Illness Care

Despite the huge and growing burden of chronic disease, which is estimated to account for 75% of all primary care visits (http://medicaleconomics.modern-medicine.com/medical-economics/news/chronic-disease-growing-challenge-pcps?page=full), the current healthcare system is not set up to promote adherence to chronic illness care. The most important *systems-related factors* currently limiting provision of chronic illness care appear to be:

- Lack of time during routine follow-up healthcare visits to address adherence and related issues like psychosocial adjustment
- Lack of physician training in assessment of adherence and health promotion strategies
- Limited dissemination of empirically-supported interventions for adherence difficulties
- Limited availability (or utilization) of behavioral health specialists with expertise in adherence
- Lack of reimbursement for preventive services and adherence interventions
- Lack of an *integrated approach* to promoting adherence and managing nonadherence

Lack of Time   Most medical professionals simply have too little time to complete assessment of adherence and psychosocial risk in children with chronic illness. A survey of over 2000 parents found that nearly 80% reported spending less than 20 min with their healthcare provider during well child visits, and a third (33.6%) reported spending less than 10 min. Not surprisingly, longer visits were associated with significantly more psychosocial risk assessment and family-centered care (Halfon et al. 2011). Halfon et al. concluded that current visit times are often insufficient to meet American Academy of Pediatrics guidelines for provision of preventive (well) healthcare.

Managing a child's chronic illness in this context can be even more challenging (Drotar et al. 2010). Studies of adults indicate that even basic aspects of chronic disease care are often neglected. For example, a study of adults with type 2 diabetes found that medical residents spent an average of only 5 min discussing diabetes with these patients, which was too little time to address hemoglobin A1c levels in the majority (60%) of cases; and only 15% of patients in poor glycemic control had their regimens adjusted (Barnes et al. 2004).

Lack of Training   Unfortunately, many healthcare professionals receive little training in chronic illness management and in other facets of care that have been shown to promote treatment adherence. One recent survey of pediatric residency program directors in adolescent medicine (Fox et al. 2010) found that only about 4 in 10 programs reported good coverage of chronic illness management in either formal education or clinical training.

The same study (Fox et al. 2010) also found minimal coverage of behavioral health, noting that "in most programs, numerous adolescent health topics, particularly those related to mental and behavioral health, are covered only somewhat or not covered at all" (p. 170). Primary care providers also report having limited knowledge of behavioral health and express concern that they do not have the training to allow them to manage psychosocial concerns in their patient (Varni et al. 2005).

Many medical schools now incorporate training in physician-patient communication skills in recognition of research demonstrating that effective provider communication results in significantly improved patient adherence (Zolnierek and DiMatteo 2009). This is an important development. One concern, however, is that this training tends to occur during the first 2 years of medical school, despite the fact that most patient contact occurs thereafter, potentially limiting its impact on actual provider behavior (Levinson et al. 2010). There are some training program for practicing physicians, but these remain relatively limited in scope to date.

Finally, many healthcare providers do not recognize adherence difficulties in their patients (Brown and Bussell 2011), at least not until the problem has become so big as to be impossible to miss. Utilization of the many evidence-based assessment tools (Quittner et al. 2008) by pediatricians and primary care physicians is quite limited. Screening for nonadherence and potentially contributory psychosocial problems is discussed in Chap. 12.

Moreover, when adherence problems *are* uncovered, many providers will assume that the patient or family lacks the knowledge or understanding for effective disease management, and so will focus on providing additional education. Unfortunately, educational approaches by themselves have very little effect on nonadherence (Chap. 4), with meta-analyses showing overall effect sizes for educational interventions in the small-to-negligible range (Graves et al. 2010; Kahana et al. 2008). As mentioned above, behavioral health training for medical providers is quite limited, so adherence problems are often not recognized as the behavioral issue that they almost always are. At the same time, many providers report being uncomfortable with asking about patients' behavioral and psychological functioning, or they lack the time to do so (Detmar et al. 2001; Levinson and Roter 1995; Maguire et al. 1996).

Limited Dissemination and Availability of Behavioral Health Services As we discuss in Chap. 4, we now have very effective interventions for treating nonadherence (Kahana et al. 2008) that also result in demonstrated improvements in children's health (Graves et al. 2010). These interventions have been developed by, and designed for, psychologists and other professionals with expertise in behavioral health. However, a number of barriers currently limit the dissemination of evidence-based interventions for pediatric nonadherence.

It is often noted that behavioral health services—i.e., the services of health psychologists and similarly trained professionals—are limited (e.g., Kazak 2006). This may be true in rural areas, but most major medical centers have some availability of behavioral health services. In some respects this lack may be more apparent than real. Many primary care providers say that they simply do not know where to refer pediatric patients with mental health concerns (Varni et al. 2005). Current movements to include mental and behavioral health professionals in primary care under the umbrella of the family-centered medical home (Medical Home Initiatives for Children With Special Needs Project Advisory Committee, and American Academy of Pediatrics 2002) may go a long way toward alleviating this problem of access.

It also appears that there is a limited awareness of the role psychologists can play in adherence promotion. Indeed, one prominent researcher has noted

> A caveat is that nonadherence per se is not considered a psychiatric disorder. Mental health providers are best equipped to handle mental health disorders (which are sometimes related to nonadherence) but do not necessarily have expertise in handling nonadherence per se. (Shemesh et al 2010)

As we discuss in a subsequent chapter, psychologists' expertise in behavior and behavior change is of critical importance to managing complex and difficult cases of nonadherence. We will also make the case for an expanded role in risk screening and prevention.

There are other barriers to accessing psychological services that in turn severely limit the availability of effective, evidence-based interventions for the patients who need them. One important barrier is the stigma (or perceived stigma) of seeing a psychologist (Schwartz et al. 2011). When referred to a pediatric psychologist, many families will say something like, "I'm not crazy" and refuse care. Helping families understand that most behavioral health psychological interventions are *specifically focused* on adherence and other health-related behaviors can make the difference in whether families follow-up for recommended care.

Lack of Reimbursement Reimbursement for behavioral and psychological services focused on adherence does remain an issue. Health and Behavior CPT codes have been written precisely to allow psychologists to provide and get reimbursed for behavioral health services, such as interventions to promote adherence (Noll and Fischer 2004), although these codes have not been implemented by Medicare/ Medicaid in every state, limiting their availability. (We cannot bill for H&B codes in our own state, Texas.)

Lack of an Integrated Approach Efforts at improving adherence have further been limited by a tendency for interventions to focus on a single barrier or contributing factor to nonadherence to the exclusion of others. As we discuss in the next section, many different factors can contribute to suboptimal adherence. Multisystemic interventions (see Chap. 4) are a promising step toward a more encompassing approach.

Nonadherence is a Multi-Factorial Problem

> Adherence is a multidimensional phenomenon determined by the interplay of five sets of factors, here termed "dimensions", of which patient-related factors are just one determinant....
> The common belief that patients are solely responsible for taking their treatment is misleading and most often reflects a misunderstanding of how other factors affect people's behavior and capacity to adhere to their treatment.—Sabate 2003

Fig. 1.1 WHO five dimensions of adherence. (Sabate 2003)

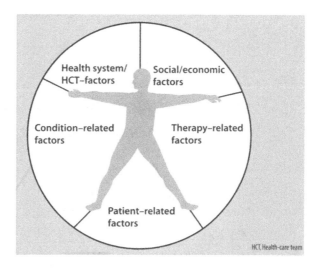

Many factors play into adherence success or failure. The World Health Organization proposed a five-factor model of adherence comprised of (1) social and economic factors, (2) healthcare team and health system factors, (3) condition-related factors, (4) therapy (or treatment)-related factors, and (5) patient-related factors (Fig. 1.1). The five-factor model was developed to characterize adherence in adults; as a result it omits a critical dimension of pediatric adherence, namely *parenting*.

De Civita and Dobkin's (2004) *triadic partnership model* better captures this aspect of pediatric adherence. This model conceives of adherence as resulting from transactions between the child, the caregiver(s), and the medical team, that are in turn influenced by development and contextual characteristics and by changes in disease course. A simplified depiction of the model is presented in Fig. 1.2. We will return to this conceptualization at the end of this book. For now, though, we wish to stress that this model will guide much of how we present our "snapshot from the field" of pediatric adherence. We will focus on transactions between the child, parents, and healthcare providers when discussing barriers and facilitators of adherence (Chap. 3), effective interventions (Chap. 4), developmental effects (e.g., adherence in adolescence; Chaps. 5 and 6), and vulnerable populations and health disparities (Chaps. 8 and 9).

In our view, the triadic partnership can be conceived of as a distinct *microsystem* within Bronfenbrenner's (1979) ecological systems theory that interacts with other microsystems (e.g., the healthcare system, school) within the broader society and culture.

Larger Societal Issues also Affect Adherence

Finally, it is important to recognize the disproportionate burden and impact of chronic illness on minorities and impoverished families. Children from poor and minority families are much more likely to have a chronic illness such as asthma or type 2 diabetes, are less likely to have the resources and access to quality care

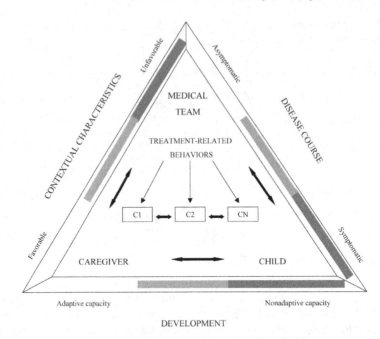

Fig. 1.2 The triadic partnership model. After De Civita and Dobkin (2004)

necessary to manage the illness effectively, and tend to have substantially worse adherence and illness control (Adler et al. 1994). It is quite possible that some of the lack of progress in reducing rates of nonadherence reflects these larger societal issues of poverty and racial/ethnic disenfranchisement. These are complex issues that are discussed in detail in Chaps. 8 and 9, but we do wish to suggest here that we do believe there may be feasible ways to promote better adherence even in these most vulnerable populations.

Summary

The complexities surrounding adherence and nonadherence can make the problem feel unwieldy. Of course, things become more manageable when viewed from the perspective of helping the individual patient struggling with adherence, for whom there are effective interventions. Even so, nonadherence can be a very frustrating problem for healthcare professionals.

One challenge is that the multi-factorial nature of nonadherence makes it something like the hydra of Greek myth—once you cut off one head, two more spring up in its place. A potential solution to this dilemma is to develop *systems-wide* approaches that can address multiple aspects of adherence. For example, to help a teenager severely struggling with adherence to his diabetes regimen may require: working with his endocrinologist to improve communication and reduce "shame and blame" tactics that make the youth very reticent to attend clinic appointments (Wolpert and Anderson 2001); providing family therapy focused on reducing parent-child conflict over diabetes management; using electronic reminders over his cell phone as a non-intrusive way to prompt blood glucose checks; and helping the family reinstate their insurance so they can afford his insulin.

A second major challenge is that adherence problems lie on a continuum from small to large—yet even small problems can have big effects at the population level. The interventions reviewed in Chap. 4 have been designed to be implemented primarily by health psychologists, and other providers with behavioral health training such as clinical social workers. These interventions are mostly geared toward patients with more intractable adherence problems or comorbid psychosocial difficulties—i.e., the patients with the highest level of risk and need, who often require the most care and resources from their healthcare providers (Anderson 2012).

However, the bulk of patients who have some difficulty with regimen adherence may not need to see a psychologist, but might instead see sufficient benefit if their primary medical providers were better able to assess and promote adherence. Indeed, most of the calls for improving adherence focus primarily on the role of medical providers. It is actually an open empirical question whether the problem of nonadherence can be effectively addressed without more wide-scale use of specialty care provided by health psychologists, an issue that will be taken up again in Chap. 11. For now, though, it is clear that in most cases promoting adherence falls to patients' medical providers. Unfortunately, the realities of contemporary healthcare make it quite challenging for clinicians to address adherence issues in routine follow-up care, although this may change as the current healthcare system continues to evolve (Kocher et al. 2010; Koh and Sebelius 2010).

To address these two main issues—the multifactorial nature of nonadherence and its dimensional nature—we provide at the end of this book a comprehensive model for risk assessment, triage, and referral of patients struggling with adherence or at risk for nonadherence; and link this system to a tiered intervention model based on a preventive health model developed for pediatric patients (Kazak 2006).

References

Adams CD, Dreyer ML, Dinakar C, Portnoy JM. Pediatric asthma: a look at adherence from the patient and family perspective. Curr Allergy Asthma Rep. 2004;4(6):425–32.

Adler NE, Boyce T, Chesney MA, et al. Socioeconomic status and health. The challenge of the gradient. Am Psychol. 1994;49:15–24.

Anderson BJ. Who forgot? The challenges of family responsibility for adherence in vulnerable pediatric populations. Pediatrics. 2012;129(5):e1324–25.

Ashton CM, Haidet P, Paterniti DA, Collins TC, Gordon HS, O'Malley K, et al. Racial and ethnic disparities in the use of health services: bias, preferences, or poor communication? J Gen Intern Med. 2003;18(2):146–52.

Barnes CS, Ziemer DC, Miller CD, et al. Little time for diabetes management in the primary care setting. Diabetes Educ. 2004;30:126–35.

Bender B, Wambolt FS, O'Connor SL, et al. Measurement of children's asthma medication adherence by self report, mother report, canister weight, and doser CT. Ann Allergy Athmsa Immunol. 2000;85:416–21.

Bronfenbrenner U. The ecology of human development: experiments by nature and design. Cambridge: Harvard University Press; 1979.

Brown MT, Bussell JK. Medication adherence: who cares. Mayo Clin Proc. 2011;86(4):304–14.

Buchanan AL, Montepiedra G, Sirois PA, et al. Barriers to medication adherence in HIV-infected children and youth based on self- and caregiver report. Pediatrics. 2012;129(5):e1244–51.

Cassell EJ. Illness and disease. Hastings Cent Rep. 1976;6(2);27–37.

Charach A, Yeung E, Volpe T, Goodale T, dosReis S. Exploring stimulant treatment in ADHD: narratives of young adolescents and their parents. BMC Psychiatry. 2014;14:110.

Chesney M. Adherence to HAART regimens. AIDS Patient Care STDS. 2003;17(4):169–77.

De Civita M, Dobkin PL Pediatric adherence as a multidimensional and dynamic construct, involving a triadic partnership. J Ped Psychol. 2004;29:157–69.

Detmar SB, Muller MJ, Wever LDV, Schornagel JH, Aaronson NK. Patient-physician communication during outpatient palliative treatment visits. JAMA. 2001;285:1351–57.

DiMatteo MR. Variations in patients' adherence to medical recommendations: a quantitative review of 50 years of research. Med Care. 2004;42:200–9.

Dobbels F, Ruppar T, De Geest S, Decorte A., Van Damme-Lombaerts, Fine RN. Adherence to the immunosuppressive regimen in pediatric kidney transplant recipients: a systematic review. Pediatr Transplant. 2010;5:603–13.

Drotar D, Crawford P, Bonner M. Collaborative decision making and treatment adherence promotion in the management of pediatric chronic illness. Patient Intell. 2010;2:1–7.

Epstein RM, Street RL. The values and value of patient-centered care. Ann Fam Med. 2011;9:100–3.

Fox H, McManus M, Klein J, Diaz A, Elster A, Felice M, Kaplan D, Wibbelsman C, Wilson J: Adolescent Medicine training in pediatric residency programs. Pediatrics. 2010;125(1):165–72.

Gadkari AS, McHorney CA. Unintentional non-adherence to chronic prescription medications: how unintentional is it really? BMC Health Serv Res. 2012;12(1):98.

Gerrard M, Gibbons FX, Houlihan AE, Stock ML, Pomery EA. A dual-process approach to health risk decision-making: the prototype-willingness model. Dev Rev. 2008;28:29–61.

Gibbons FX. Intention, expectation, and willingness 2008. http://cancercontrol.cancer.gov/BRP/constructs/intent-expect-willingness/iew4.html. Accessed 12 Mar 2015.

Gibbons FX, Gerrard M. Health images and their effects on health behavior. In: Buunk BP, Gibbons FX, editors, Health, coping, and well-being: perspectives from social comparison theory. Mahwah: Lawrence Erlbaum Associates, Publishers; 1997. pp. 63–94.

Glasgow RM. Perceived barriers to self-management and preventive behaviors 2008. http://cancercontrol.cancer.gov/BRP/constructs/barriers/index.html. Accessed 12 Mar 2015.

Graves MM, Roberts MC, Rapoff M, Boyer A. The efficacy of adherence interventions for chronically ill children: a meta-analytic review. J Pediatr Psychol. 2010;35:368–82.

Halfon N, Stevens GD, Larson K, Olson LM. Duration of a well-child visit: association with content, family-centeredness, and satisfaction. Pediatrics. 2011;128:657–64. doi:10.1542/peds.2011-0586.

Haynes RB. Interventions for helping patients to follow prescriptions for medications. Cochrane Database Syst Rev. 2001;1.

Haynes RB, Taylor DW, Sackett DL. Compliance in health care. Baltimore: Johns Hopkins University Press; 1979.

Helman CG. Disease versus illness in general practice. J R Coll Gen Pract. 1981;31:548–52.

Hood KK, Peterson CM, Rohan JM, Drotar D. Association between adherence and glycemic control in pediatric type 1 diabetes: a meta-analysis. Pediatrics. 2009;124(6):e1171–79.

Horne R, Weinman J, Barber N, Elliott R, Morgan M, Cribb A. Concordance, adherence and compliance in medicine-taking. London: NCCSDO; 2005.

Kahana S, Drotar D, Frazier T. Meta-analysis of psychological interventions to promote adherence to treatment in pediatric chronic health conditions. J Pediatr Psychol. 2008;33:590–611.

Kaufman FR, Halvorson M, Carpenter S. Association between diabetes control and visits to a multidisciplinary pediatric diabetes clinic. Pediatrics. 1999;103:948–51.

Kazak AE. Pediatric psychosocial preventative health model (PPPHM): research, practice and collaboration in pediatric family systems medicine. Fam Syst Health. 2006;24;381–95.

Kocher R, Emanuel EJ, DeParle NAM. The affordable care act and the future of clinical medicine: the opportunities and challenges. Ann Intern Med. 2010;153:536–9.

Koh HK, Sebelius KG. Promoting prevention through the affordable care act. N Engl J Med 2010;363:1296–9.

La Greca AM, Bearman KJ. If an apple a day keeps the doctor away, why is adherence so hard? J Pediatr Psychol. 2001;26:279–82.

Laffel L, Brackett J, Ho J, Anderson BJ. Changing the process of diabetes care improves metabolic outcomes and reduces hospitalizations. Qual Manage Health Care. 1998;6:53–62.

Levinson W, Roter D. Physicians' psychosocial beliefs correlate with their patient communication skills. J Gen Intern Med. 1995;10:375–9.

Levinson W, Lesser CS, Epstein RM. Developing physician communication skills for patient-centered care. Health Aff. 2010;29(7):1310–18.

Lorig KR, Holman H. Self-management education: history, definition, outcomes, and mechanisms. Ann Behav Med. 2003;26:1–7.

Maguire P, Faulkner A, Booth K, Elliott C, Hillier V. Helping cancer patients disclose their concerns. Eur J Cancer. 1996;32A(1):78–81.

Maldonado M, Chong E, Oehl M, Balasubramanyam A. Economic impact of diabetic ketoacidosis in a multiethnic indigent population: analysis of costs based on the precipitating cause. Diabetes Care. 2003;26:1265–69.

Medical Home Initiatives for Children With Special Needs Project Advisory Committee. American academy of pediatrics. The medical home. Pediatrics. 2002;110(1 Pt 1):184–6.

Modi AC, Pai AL, Hommel KA, et al. Pediatric self-management: a framework for research, practice, and policy. Pediatrics. 2012;129:e473–85.

Noll R, Fischer M. Commentary: health and behavior CPT codes: an opportunity to revolutionize reimbursement in pediatric psychology. J Pediatr Psychol. 2004;29;571–8.

Oliva M, Singh TP, Gauvreau K, VanderPluym CJ, Bastardi HJ, Almond CS. Impact of medication non-adherence on survival after pediatric heart transplantation in the USA. J Heart Lung Transplant. 2013;32:881–8.

Quittner AL, Modi AC, Lemanek KL, Ievers-Landis CE, Rapoff MA. Evidence-based assessment of adherence to medical treatments in pediatric psychology. J Pediatr Psychol. 2008;33:916–36.

Penza-Clyve SM, Mansell C, McQuaid EL. Why don't children take their asthma medications? A qualitative analysis of children's perspectives on adherence. Journal of Asthma 2004;41:189–97.

Rapoff MA. Adherence to pediatric medical regimens. 2nd ed. New York: Springer; 2010.

Rapoff MA, Barnard MU. Compliance with pediatric medical regimens. In: Cramer JA, Spilker B, editors. Patient compliance in medical practice and clinical trials. New York: Raven; 1991. pp. 73–98.

Roter DL, Stewart M, Putnam SM, Lipkin M, Stiles W, Inui TS. Communication styles of primary care physicians. JAMA. 1997;277:350–6.

Sabate, E. Adherence to long-term therapies: evidence for action. Geneva: World Health Organization; 2003.

Santer et al. Treatment non-adherence in pediatric long-term medical conditions: systematic review and synthesis of qualitative studies of caregivers' views. BMC Pediatr. 2014;14:63.

Schwartz DD, Cline VD, Hansen J, Axelrad ME, Anderson BJ. Early risk factors for nonadherence in pediatric type 1 diabetes: a review of the recent literature. Curr Diabetes Rev. 2010;6:167–83.

Schwartz DD, Cline VD, Axelrad ME, Anderson BJ. Feasibility, acceptability, and predictive validity of a psychosocial screening program for children and youth newly diagnosed with Type 1 diabetes. Diabetes Care. 2011;34:326–31.

Schwartz D, Axelrad M, Anderson B. Psychosocial risk screening of children newly diagnosed with type 1 diabetes: a training toolkit for healthcare professionals. MedEdPORTAL; 2013. www.mededportal.org/publication/9643. Accessed 12 Mar 2015.

Shemesh E. Non-adherence to medications following pediatric liver transplantation. Pediatr Transplant. 2004;8:600–5.

Shemesh E, Annunziato RA, Arnon R, Miloh T, Kerkar N. Adherence to medical recommendations and transition to adult services in pediatric transplant recipients. Curr Opin Organ Transplant. 2010;15:288–92.

Simoni JM, Montgomery A, Martin E, New M, Demas PA, Rana S. Adherence to antiretroviral therapy for pediatric HIV infection: a qualitative systematic review with recommendations for research and clinical management. Pediatrics. 2007;119:e1371–83.

Stark L. Introduction to the special issue on adherence in pediatric medical conditions. J Pediatr Psychol. 2013;38:589–94.

Street RL, O'Malley KJ, Cooper LA, Haidet P. Understanding concordance in patient-physician relationships: personal and ethnic dimensions of shared identity. Ann Fam Med. 2008;6:198–205.

Svoren B, Butler D, Levine B, Anderson B, Laffel L. Reducing acute adverse outcomes in youth with type 1 diabetes mellitus: a randomized controlled trial. Pediatrics. 2003;112:914–22.

Van Cleave J, Gortmaker SL, Perrin JM. Dynamics of obesity and chronic health conditions among children and youth. JAMA. 2010;303:623–30.

van Es SM, le Coq EM, Brownwert AI, et al. Adherence-related behavior in adolescents with asthma: results from focus group interviews. J Asthma. 1998;35:637–46.

Varni J, Burwinkle T, Lane M. Health-related quality of life measurement in pediatric clinical practice: an appraisal and precept for future research and application. Health Qual Life Outcomes. 2005;3:1–9.

Viswanathan M, Golin CE, Jones CD, Ashok M, Blalock S, Wines RCM, Coker-Schwimmer EJL, Grodensky CA, Rosen DL, Yuen A, Sista P, Lohr KN. Medication adherence interventions: comparative effectiveness. closing the quality gap: revisiting the state of the science. Evidence report No. 208. (Prepared by RTI International–University of North Carolina Evidence-based Practice Center under Contract No. 290-2007-10056-I.) AHRQ Publication No. 12-E010-EF. Rockville, MD: Agency for Healthcare Research and Quality. September 2012. www.effective-healthcare.ahrq.gov/reports/final.cfm.

Winkley K, Ismail K, Landau S, Eisler I. Psychological interventions to improve glycaemic control in patients with type 1 diabetes: systematic review and meta-analysis of randomised controlled trials. BMJ. 2006;333(7558):65.

Wolpert HA, Anderson BJ. Management of diabetes: are doctors framing the benefits from the wrong perspective? BMJ. 2001;323:994–6.

Wolfsdorf J, Craig ME, Daneman D, Dunger D, Edge J, Lee W, Rosenbloom A, Sperling M, Hanas R. Diabetic ketoacidosis in children and adolescents with diabetes. Pediatr Diabetes. 2009;10:118–33.

Wroe AL, Intentional and unintentional nonadherence: a study of decision making. J behav med. 2002;25(4):355–72.

Zolnierek KBH, DiMatteo MR. Physician communication and patient adherence to treatment: a meta-analysis. Med Care. 2009;47:826–34.

Chapter 2
Conceptualizing Adherence

Abstract In this chapter we review theoretical constructs that have proved crucial to our thinking and approach to pediatric adherence. This is not meant to be a comprehensive review of current theories, but a selective examination of some key points. Constructs familiar from the adult literature are considered from the perspective of family-centered care, which entails recognition of the different roles the family plays in helping manage a child's chronic illness. In later chapters these key concepts will further inform discussion of the roles of parents and healthcare providers in fostering children's adherence and eventual attainment of autonomous and independent self-care skills.

Theories are explanatory systems that provide a way to bring together diverse aspects of a subject in a way that can help foster understanding of the big picture. They "organize experience, generate inferences, guide learning, and influence behavior and social interactions" (Gelman and Legare 2011). Many parents (and clinicians) are influenced by "folk theories" of why people do or do not adhere to their medical regimen—unexamined and untested beliefs that arise from the culture and personal experience. Theories based in science provide a corrective view to these beliefs, ground an understanding of *why* people struggle with adherence, and suggest or open ways to help improve adherence and illness management more generally.

One challenge of applying theoretical models of adherence to children is that all of the main models have been developed with adults in mind. Rapoff (2010) therefore cautioned against extrapolating conclusions about children's adherence from adult-based models. In contrast to adults, who manage an estimated 95–99 % of their own chronic illness care themselves (Funnell 2000), children do not manage illness independently. Pediatric illness management is complicated by the fact that multiple players are involved, by developmental changes that can make adherence a moving target, and by interactions between development and parenting, which has to be adapted accordingly. In addition, complexities arise in the interaction between the family and their healthcare providers. For example, in working with a teen and her parents, it can be difficult to know who the provider should speak with about which health-related issues.

When children are younger, parents have sole responsibility for illness management, but as the child gets older, management responsibility shifts increasingly to

© Springer International Publishing Switzerland 2015

D. D. Schwartz, M. E. Axelrad, *Healthcare Partnerships for Pediatric Adherence,*
SpringerBriefs in Public Health, DOI 10.1007/978-3-319-13668-4_2

the child. Pediatric adherence can therefore be seen as involving a *transaction* between parent and child, in which child behavior and parenting practices influence
each other reciprocally (Sameroff 2009). The ways in which parents and their children interact has a tremendous impact on whether and how well the child's illness
is managed.

The transactional nature of pediatric adherence is one of the main complications
in trying to extrapolate from adult models and concepts of adherence. Adult models
of health behavior and adherence highlight concepts such as *beliefs, goals, intentions*, and *motivation* as important drivers of adherence behavior, yet when applied
to pediatrics, the question repeatedly arises of *whose* beliefs, goals, etc. should be
the focus of consideration—the child's or the parent's (Schwartz and Drotar 2006)?
Or consider the model of *patient-centered care*, which has become one of the cor-
nerstones of modern illness management, within which "patients are known as persons in context of their own social worlds, listened to, informed, respected, and
involved in their care—and their wishes are honored (but not mindlessly enacted)
during their health care journey" (Epstein and Street 2011). How can a provider be
patient-centered in this sense with a 4-year old, or even a 10- or 12-year old child?
Whose wishes are to be honored?

The solution is that, in pediatrics, it is not enough to be patient-centered; instead,
care must be *family-centered*. This means taking both child and parent perspectives
into account. But what should be done when parent and child perspectives diverge,
when the parent wants one thing and the child another? How are parent-child differences in beliefs, goals, and values to be navigated and negotiated? Obviously development plays a role. Early in development, the parent perspective dominates, but
over time the child perspective becomes increasingly important, eventually eclips-
ing the parent at the time of transition into adulthood. Even so, this leaves open a
long stretch of developmental time—let's call it adolescence—when there can be
as much conflict as cooperation, and goals may clash (Schwartz and Drotar 2006).
What should be done when parent and child perspectives diverge, when the parent
wants one thing and the child another?

In the sections that follow, we selectively review conceptual models of important
factors that underlie adherence. Sections are organized to roughly follow the process of adaptation individuals often go through from disease diagnosis to initiation
of health-related behaviors (Fig. 2.1). We first review *stress/and coping* models that
describe how individuals adapt to a new disease. We then discuss the importance of
disease- and treatment-related *knowledge* as a necessary foundation for illness management, and the ways in which *health beliefs* of both patient and parent affect their
understanding and utilization of their knowledge. Health beliefs in turn influence
the *goals* individuals set for themselves, which serve as action plans for subsequent
adherence behaviors. *Self-regulation* models describe the capabilities that underlie
goal-striving—namely, the individual's ability to exert self-control such that future
goals can be attained. These factors in turn help determine a person's underlying
motivation for engaging in adherence behaviors that may have no immediate benefits but are critical for long-term health.

Fig. 2.1 Hypothetical model
of the process of adapta-
tion, from initial coping to
adherence

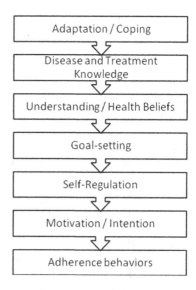

Stress and Coping Models of Illness Adaptation

When a child is first diagnosed with a chronic illness, it is often a shock to the family; and in many cases diagnosis is experienced as traumatic, especially if the caregiver or child fears the child may die or be seriously harmed. High rates of post-traumatic stress symptoms have been reported in parents of children diagnosed with cancer (Kazak et al. 1998) and type 1 diabetes (Cline et al. 2011; Landolt et al. 2002). Less severely, about one in three children develop a diagnosable adjustment disorder at diagnosis (Cameron et al. 2007).

For most children with a chronic illness and their families, the shock dissipates but a sense of chronic stress remains. As we noted in the Introduction, many illnesses require complex and intrusive daily management; others, such as asthma and sickle cell disease, have recurrent (and sometimes unpredictable) symptom flares; and still others (e.g., cystic fibrosis) result in substantial functional limitations and disability.

The recognition that a chronic illness becomes a chronic stressor to which the child and family adapt is at the core of *stress and coping models* of illness adjustment (e.g., Thompson and Gustafson 1996; Wallander and Varni 1998). Also important is the idea that the condition requires "continual readjustment" and "repeatedly interfere[s] with the adequate performance of ordinary role-related activities" (Wallander and Varni 1998). Adjustment requires the child and family to manage emotional responses, consider social implications, and martial resources both within and outside the family for managing the disease and maintaining (or returning) to "life as normal" as far as possible. It also requires children and families to "change and reprioritize … goals in order to incorporate new goals related to [illness] management" (Schwartz and Drotar 2006).

Children and their families draw on their resources to cope with illness. In Wallander and Varni's (1998) model, these so-called *resilience factors* include a person's competence and skills, family environment, social support, practical resources, and "stress-processing factors such as cognitive appraisal and coping strategies." At the same time, pre-existing or co-existing *risk factors* interfere with or complicate children's and families' abilities to cope and manage the illness. Important risk factors include disease-related disability, reduced ability to complete activities of daily living, and psychosocial stressors (Wallander and Varni 1998). An important contribution of stress and coping models has been to identify modifiable risk factors that can be targeted for intervention.

More recent models of coping with chronic illness have focused on the dimension of *control* (Compas et al. 2012). *Primary control* (or active coping) refers to efforts to change the source of stress or one's reactions to it, whereas *secondary control* refers to efforts to accommodate to the stressor. *Disengagement* or passive coping refers to avoidance or lack of any coping attempts (Rudolph et al. 1995). Not surprisingly, disengagement or avoidance coping has been associated with poorer adherence (e.g., Reid et al. 1994).

In a recent review, Compas et al. (2012) noted that secondary coping has the strongest support in terms of child adjustment to illness, and they suggested that the uncontrollable nature of many illnesses requires adaptation rather than active attempts to control the disease. This finding is consistent with the burnout often seen among children and youth who attempt to maintain tight illness control and sheds some light on why children and youth with better adherence sometimes have worse psychosocial adjustment. It may also shed light on a point made over a decade ago by La Greca and Bearman (2001): "What may appear to be 'nonadherence' to a health care professional may actually be the family's way of adapting the regimen to accommodate the child's quality of life." In other words, poor adherence when an illness is especially difficult to control may sometimes be the most effective coping strategy, at least in terms of maximizing immediate quality of life. The fact that adherence and quality of life are often at odds may be the most challenging aspect of maintaining good illness control. As noted by Schwartz and Drotar (2006) in discussing a hypothetical youth with diabetes, "if prioritizing and working towards her health-related goals compromises her ability to pursue and achieve other personally salient goals, then she may feel that her [chronic health condition] is affecting her quality of life and adaptation."

Illness and Treatment Knowledge and Health Literacy

Managing a chronic illness requires a new set of knowledge and skills to carry out health behaviors correctly and consistently. As noted by many authors (e.g., Adams et al. 2004; Hood et al. 2009), medical regimens have become increasingly complex, and often stretch the abilities of patients and their families. After diagnosis, physicians and other healthcare providers focus on patient and family education, although there is some question of whether enough time is spent for families to truly learn and understand the condition and its treatment for many illnesses (Turner et al. 2009), especially as diagnosis is often a time of such high stress, which can limit parents' ability to actively engage in learning.

Health literacy has been defined as "the degree to which individuals have the capacity to obtain, process, and understand basic health information and services needed to make appropriate health decisions" (US Department of Health and Human Services 2000). Recent reviews of health literacy in the pediatric domain (Abrams et al. 2009; DeWalt and Hink 2009; Yin et al. 2009) suggest the following main points:

1. Health literacy involves a complex set of skills that include reading, math (numeracy), multimedia, problem-solving and interpretive skills.
2. Health literacy is closely associated with general literacy, and with socioeconomic and cultural factors that are themselves related to literacy (see Chap. 8)
3. Health literacy "*must be considered in terms of parents' or caregivers' health literacy as well as the children's own health literacy* (which is evolving as children grow, learn, and develop)" (Abrams et al. 2009; emphasis added)
4. Low parent health literacy is associated with worse child health outcomes, especially for younger children
5. Low health literacy among adolescents is associated with greater general risk-taking behavior but there is no evidence of an association with worse adherence
6. Overall, low health literacy is associated with worse adherence, BUT
7. Interventions to improve health literacy have been shown to improve health *knowledge* but at best have weak and indirect effects on health *behavior*

Regarding the last point above, a recent meta-analysis of interventions for pediatric nonadherence reported negligible-to-small effect sizes for education-only interventions ($d=0.16$, 95 % CI $= 0.10$–0.22; Kahana et al. 2008). Education *is* an important component of interventions for adherence, however. A second meta-analysis (Graves et al. 2010) found that interventions that combined educational with behavioral approaches had more potent effects on health outcomes ($d=0.74$, 95 % CI $= 0.55$–0.94) than either type of approach alone ($d=0.16$, 95 % CI $= 0.02$–0.30). Moreover, Graves et. found that educational approaches resulted in better long-term health outcomes on follow-up. Taken together, these findings support the notion that education is necessary but not sufficient for adherence to medical recommendations (DeWalt and Hink 2009).

It is also important to recognize that knowledge is different from the ability to use that knowledge successfully. For example, caregivers in the National Cooperative Inner-City Asthma Study demonstrated good knowledge of asthma (M $= 84$ % correct answers on an asthma information quiz), but when presented with hypothetical problem situations most offered at least one solution that was "potentially dangerous or maladaptive" (Wade et al. 1997). Interventions that focus on teaching illness-specific problem-solving skills (e.g., Grey and Berry 2004) are likely to be more effective than interventions focused on increasing knowledge.

Many factors play into families' understanding of disease and illness. Healthcare providers are used to taking for granted the empirical basis for most of what they do—clinical guidelines and best practice recommendations are based, to the degree possible, on the best available scientific evidence. Many laypeople do not think this way, however. It must be acknowledged that there is a lot of distrust of medicine and "Big Pharma." For example, a recent Pew poll found that only one quarter of U.S. adults have a lot of confidence that new medicines have been carefully tested before being made available to the public, half had "some" confidence, while the last quarter had little to no confidence (http://www.pewforum.org/2013/08/06/chapter-4-views-about-todays-medical-treatments-and-advances/). Many people use alternative therapies despite the lack of an empirical basis. A National Science Foundation survey from 2001 found that 88% of respondents agreed that "there are some good ways of treating sickness that medical science does not recognize" (Science and Technology: Public Attitudes and Public Understanding; http://www.nsf.gov/statistics/seind02/c7/c7s5.htm#c7s5l2a), and all indications are that use of alternative therapies has only increased since that time.

Health Beliefs

Adjustment and coping attempts and adherence all rely on the child and family's beliefs about the illness, its controllability, treatment, and their own capabilities. According to Helman (1981) in a classic article:

Faced with an episode of ill-health, patients try to explain what has happened, why it has happened and decide what to do about it. The shaping of the illness and the behavior of the patient—and of those around him—will depend on the answers to six questions:

• What has happened?
• Why has it happened?
• Why to me?
• Why now?
• What would happen if nothing was done about it?
• What should I do about it or whom should I consult for further help?

How the questions are answered, and the behavior that follows, constitutes a 'folk model of illness'.

In other words, patients (and their families) will attempt to come to an understanding of what the illness is and what it means to them.

The *Health Belief Model* (HBM; e.g., Janz and Becker 1984) posits that people's adherence will be influenced by their beliefs that the illness poses a true threat to their health, that the treatment is effective and its benefits outweigh its costs, and they are capable of doing what they need to do to manage the illness. The HBM has a substantial amount of empirical support in the adult literature and has been one of the most influential theories of health-related behavior. But to the degree that pediatric adherence results from an interaction between the child and his/her caregivers, the question arises, *whose* health beliefs should be considered (La Greca and Mackey 2009)? This question is especially important as child and parent health beliefs are not always correlated (Charron-Prochownik et al. 1993).

Parent Beliefs Parent health beliefs have a significant impact on children's illness management. Adherence tends to be poor when parents are concerned about medication safety or side-effects. One study of children with asthma and their parents looked at the difference between parents' perceived necessity of medication and their concerns about adverse effects or dependency (Kelly et al. 2007). Adherence increased as the differential between perceived need and concern widened, and adherence was lowest when concerns exceeded perceived necessity. Minority parents were more likely to have concerns about medication, as were parents who reported using alternative therapies. An even more dramatic demonstration of the importance of parent beliefs can be seen in the recent recurrence of diseases such as measles (declared to be eradicated in the U.S. in 2000) due to caregivers' erroneous beliefs about the safety of vaccines (Diekema 2012).

It should also be kept in mind that most children have multiple caregivers, not all of whom may agree about the meaning of the illness or importance of treatment. For example, we often hear anecdotal reports of multigenerational families in which a grandparent undermines the parent's attempts to manage a child's illness by expressing doubt about the need for the prescribed treatment, or a preference for a more traditional alternative medicine approach.

Child/youth beliefs The relation between children's health beliefs and adherence is much less clear. A systematic review of the relation between children and youth's health beliefs and adherence (Haller et al. 2008) found conflicting results, with about half of studies showing an association and half showing no association. Methodological differences may account for some the discrepancies, but as the authors note, "Unmeasured factors such as parents' role in affecting adherence behaviors more than beliefs may potentially explain this difference."

Indeed, few studies have examined both child and parent health beliefs and their relation to adherence within a single study. Bush and Iannotti (1990) adapted the health belief model for children (the Children's Health Belief Model) and used the model to predict children's (age 8–14 years) expected medicine use for common (acute) health problems. They first examined child health-belief predictors and then repeated the analysis entering caregiver variables, thus accounting for the effect of caregiver beliefs. Surprisingly, caregiver beliefs accounted only for a small (although statistically significant) amount of additional variance, although it should be noted that the outcome was *expected* medication use, not actual use. (They could not measure actual use because they used a sample of children without chronic illness requiring regular medication management.) It seems plausible if not likely that parents' beliefs would have a much stronger effect on whether medicines are actually taken or not.

Studies of youth with type 1 diabetes have generally shown positive effects of youth health-beliefs on adherence (although see Urquhart et al. 2002). Skinner and colleagues have consistently found relations between perceived treatment effectiveness and better diabetes self-care (diet, exercise, blood glucose monitoring, and insulin administration; Skinner and Hampson 1998; Skinner and Hampson 2001; Skinner et al. 2002). Perceived threat of diabetes has also been found to be associated with better adherence (Skinner et al. 2002), but possibly only when the costs of following the diabetes regimen are seen as low (Bond et al. 1992). Interestingly, Bond et al. found that metabolic control was worst when perceived threat and perceived cost were both high, suggesting that perceived threat may be a risk factor for poor illness control when youth struggle with management tasks. Studies of youth with asthma have also generally shown positive effects of health-beliefs in the expected directions (Buston and Wood 2000; Rich et al. 2002; Zebracki and Drotar 2004).

Many of the studies examining health beliefs in children have methodological limitations (Haller et al. 2008), especially regarding differences in measurement of the relevant constructs (Rapoff 2010). A promising measure of youth health beliefs is the Beliefs About Medication Scale (BAMS; Riekert and Drotar 2002), a 59-item scale that assesses a number of important constructs of the HBM: Perceived Threat (severity and susceptibility), Positive Outcome Expectancy (i.e., benefits), Negative Outcome Expectancy (i.e., barriers), and Intent. In the validation study of 133 adolescents with asthma, HIV, or inflammatory bowel disease, the BAMS accounted for 22 % of the variance in self-reported medication adherence. Three subscales were positively correlated with adherence and the fourth approached significance. A shorter version of the scale has also been developed to assess caregiver beliefs (Naar-King et al. 2006) and presumably could be re-adapted for use with children.

Health beliefs, as measured by the constructs of the HBM, may not be good predictors of adherence or illness control for minorities, although few studies have examined this directly. Patino et al (Patino et al. 2005) found no relation between health beliefs and adherence or glycemic control in a sample of youth with a relatively high proportion of minorities (Black and Hispanic youth). However, they did find that perceived susceptibility to diabetes was much higher and perceived severity of the illness was lower compared to the findings reported by Bond et al. (1992), suggesting that this sample saw themselves as more vulnerable but perceived the consequences of diabetes as less bad.

Overall, research findings indicate that both parent and youth health beliefs have an effect on children's adherence. Studies are needed that examine the concordance between parent and child health-beliefs and their effect on illness management. In line with this, a recent study by Herge et al. (2012) found that higher concurrent youth and parent self-efficacy for diabetes was associated with better adherence. Better understanding of health beliefs may open up new avenues for intervention, although to date interventions that have changed health beliefs have had minimal impact on adherence behavior (Strecher and Rosenstock 1997).

Goal Setting

Health beliefs strongly influence the goals people set for themselves (or for their children, or for their patients), and goals in turn drive *intentions*, or the plans and effort expended in the pursuit of goal attainment (Ajzen 1991, 1996). Intentions are seen as proximal indicators of a person's readiness to perform a behavior (Ajzen 2005) and have been shown to account for 20–30 % of the variance in health behavior in adults (Gibbons 2008).

Goal-setting is often the first step in developing a plan for behavior change. For example, a physician will set glycemic goals for a child with newly diagnosed diabetes, and an overweight youth will set weight-related goals for himself. More proximal behavioral goals in these examples might be determining the number of glucose checks the first child performs, and setting up a walking schedule and dietary targets for the second child.

However, in line with the theme of this book, goal-setting is complicated by involving multiple actors. Goal discrepancies between the child, parent(s), and healthcare providers are common. Children and their parents often have competing goals—parents tend to be more focused on illness management, whereas children focus on immediate quality of life, such as their social lives, school performance, and extracurricular activities. Health-related goal setting may place pressure on a child to alter her standards for herself in other areas of her life, such as "not having to be the best soccer player; not having to get As on every test" (Schwartz and Drotar 2006). As one can imagine, this sort of reorientation of goals and standards can entail a significant sense of loss for the child. Goal-discrepancies between parents also occur.

Children and families also may have different goals from healthcare providers. In general, healthcare providers see disease management as the primary goal, whereas families will often prioritize goals "to maintain normalcy and enhance well-being" in the family (Rehm and Franck 2000).

Some examples of differing goals between patients, parents, and healthcare providers include:

- A parent does not want a 9-year old child to know she may be infertile as a result of treatment
- A parent wishes her diabetic child to have an insulin pump for better glycemic control, whereas the child does not want to wear a device that others could see.
- A parent wants her child to have life-prolonging treatment (e.g., chest physical therapy for CF) that the child resists because of time and discomfort (Rapoff 2010)
- The parent of a child with type 1 diabetes prioritizes minimizing hypoglycemic lows whereas the physician is focused on reducing hyperglycemia (Marteau et al. 1987)
- The parents of a child with terminal illness prioritize prolonging life, whereas the medical team prioritizes minimizing suffering (Wolfe et al. 2000)

Competing views on the relative importance of different goals often result in misunderstandings and conflict—between the child and parent, or between the healthcare provider and the child or family (Schwartz and Drotar 2006), even if the provider is not aware of the conflict. As Schwartz and Drotar note, and as we discuss later in this volume, "discrepancies among invested parties will likely be minimized when there is collaboration and agreement about what goals are important and how to achieve them." Even when agreement is not achieved, simply improving communication among the relevant parties can greatly increase chances for adherence success (DiMatteo 2000).

It is also important to recognize that people often have competing goals themselves, requiring them to prioritize goals, and patients will often prioritize non-health-related goals over health-related goals. Thus "understanding and respecting patients' non-health-related goals" (Schwartz and Drotar 2006) is necessary for providers who wish to best help their patients with adherence. If providers are unaware of these competing motivations, they will be unable to discuss pros and cons with their patients. Using a motivational interviewing-style approach (see Chap. 4) may prove especially helpful here, as providers can point out the youth's own competing goals and highlight the discrepancy between them, which has been shown to help motivate behavior change. On the other hand, simply telling patients what they *should do* is very likely to backfire, as we discuss later in this chapter.

Self Regulation

Attaining health-related and adherence goals requires self-control—i.e., inhibiting an impulse to engage in some desirable behavior (such as eating a restricted food) in the interest of a goal whose benefits may be far in the future. The human animal is simply not wired to do this. Evolution predisposes us to "eat now because there may be famine tomorrow." Greater uncertainty of receiving the long-term benefit contributes to this tendency to favor immediate reward (Mischel and Ayduk 2004).

Nonetheless, people are often able to delay gratification and work toward goals that are far in the future. *Self-regulation* refers to a person's attempts to control impulses and adapt immediate behavior in the interest of attaining a long-term goal or goals (de Ridder and de Wit 2006). Models of self-regulation focus on two linked processes: setting goals, and then striving to achieve them. Successful self-regulation depends on multiple factors including having goals that are personally meaningful, a belief in one's ability to attain the goal (termed *self-efficacy*; Bandura 1997), and the skills necessary to problem-solve difficulties, overcome barriers, and cope with frustration and other emotional responses.

One may ask whether it is *self*-regulation when it is the parent who is largely in control of health management. We believe the answer is yes, as in these instances the child has to conform—to self-regulate—in response to the parent's wishes or demands. When a child is unable to do this, significant behavior problems result, often requiring intervention by a behavioral specialist. Still, as we will see, the issue

Table 2.1 Hot and cool systems of behavioral regulation. From Metcalf and Mischel 1999

Hot system	Cool system
Emotional	Cognitive
"Go"	"Know"
Simple	Complex
Reflexive	Reflective
Fast	Slow
Develops early	Develops late
Accelretaed by stress	Attenuated by stress
Stimulus control	Self-control

of *control* is critically important to self-regulation in illness management, and we will return to this issue later in this section.

It has been suggested that two different systems are involved in self-regulation: a "hot" system that responds to immediate rewards and a "cool" system involved in planful behavior necessary for obtaining delayed rewards (Metcalf and Mischel 1999; see Table 2.1). Subsequent research has shown that these systems are associated with different brain areas. Dopaminergic circuits in the limbic system are preferentially activated by decisions regarding immediate rewards (the hot system), whereas prefrontal and parietal cortical regions are associated with deliberative decision-making (the cool system) and show greater activation when decisions involve more distal rewards (McClure et al. 2004).

To the degree that adherence requires delay of immediate gratification in pursuit of long-term goals, individual differences in disparity between the hot and cool systems might be predicted to be associated with greater or lesser adherence difficulties. As we discuss in Chap. 6, a developmental lag between high (hot-system) reactivity and low (cool-system) cognitive control characterizes adolescence, a time during which adherence is often at its worst. It is highly probable that suboptimal self-regulation plays a role in the adherence difficulties of teens.

Self-regulation is viewed as an effortful process for which people have a limited capacity (Baumeister et al. 1998)—you can only expend so much effort for so long. Managing a chronic illness is likely to require persistence over a long period of time, and even with good adherence, the outcomes remain uncertain (de Ridder and de Wit 2006). These factors make maintaining a behavior over time very difficult, which can help explain why maintenance fatigue and failures are so common in chronic illness management (cf. la Greca and Bearman 2001). As discussed below, health behaviors may be easier to sustain when they reflect *intrinsic* motivations— the values and desires held by the child—than when they reflect the influence of outside motivators, including the desire to please an adult or avoid reprimands or recriminations.

Applying self-regulation frameworks to adherence is also complicated by the fact that adherence behaviors may not actually be driven by long-term goals for many or even most individuals. As de Ridder and de Wit note (p. 10), it is unclear whether people are actually "self-regulating (choosing our own goals) or are we being regulated (following doctors orders only) when we decide" to engage in a health behavior. This is a critical distinction, and it probably varies from person to person, and maybe even from behavior to behavior.

Moreover, this question has special relevance to pediatric adherence, as completion of health behaviors are often done because that's what the *parent* wants or demands—and as any parent knows, regulating your child's behavior is a very different endeavor from regulating your own (not that the latter is always easy!). However, while parent and child goals sometimes conflict outright (e.g., eating freely versus following a diet), more often there is overlap (for example, staying healthy), although it may be difficult to find that common ground if communication is poor or there is a more general simmering of underlying conflict (see Chap. 7).

Self-regulation theory accounts for a significant challenge faced by anyone who must manage a chronic illness – that is, how to manage competing motivations and impulses that run counter to long-term goals of controlling illness and maintaining health. However, current models of self-regulation are less successful in helping us understand why certain people *are* able to self-regulate in the service of goal-attainment where so many others are not (de Ridder and de Wit 2006). Individual differences certainly play a role, but so do the motivations underlying goal-directedness.

Understanding what motivates adherence, and what sustains that motivation, are concerns that cut to the core problem of pediatric adherence. Most illness management behaviors are not in themselves reinforcing, so motivation must come from somewhere else. Ideally the motivation comes from the child herself, is something that she is fully invested in and "owns," but in reality this is often not the case. Young children do not understand why they have to take a medication, or use a CPAP, or receive an injection of insulin every day. Older children may understand but still resist participating in a task they find aversive, or disruptive to their lives. In such cases parents and healthcare providers attempt to motivate the child, but as clinical experience will attest, these attempts often backfire. How can we best foster children's motivation for adherence? These questions lie at the core of *self-determination theory* (SDT), to which we now turn.

Motivation: Self Determination Theory

People are centrally concerned with **motivation**—how to move themselves or others to act. Everywhere, parents, teachers, coaches, and managers struggle with how to motivate those that they mentor, and individuals struggle to find energy, mobilize effort and persist at the tasks of life and work (http://www.selfdeterminationtheory. org/theory/)

Self Determination Theory (SDT) is a theory of motivation that focuses on the social factors and contexts that either foster or inhibit motivation (Ryan and Deci 2000). *Motivation* is defined as an influence that guides and modulates behavior based on both internal and external forces or conditions (Wilson and

Keil 2001). According to SDT, "conditions supporting the individual's experience of *autonomy, competence,* and *relatedness* are argued to foster the most volitional and high quality forms of motivation and engagement for activities" (website), including health-related activities and adherence (Ryan et al. 2008 ; Williams 2002). Motivation can either be internally-driven (by a person's own wants, needs, goals, beliefs, interests, values, etc.) or controlled by external factors (e.g., rewards, punishments, someone else's goals). Of course, the distinction between internal and external motivation is not always so clear—consider the case of a reward that a person wants badly—but the critical factor, according to SDT, is whether and to what degree the external motivator is *internalized* and taken on as a personal value or goal.

A wealth of research supports the contention that external factors such as rewards (Deci et al. 1999), threats of punishment, and surveillance all tend to *reduce* intrinsic motivation for an activity and satisfaction in its accomplishment (Deci and Ryan 2008). These approaches often result in an initial increase in the desired activity, but maintenance of the activity rarely lasts, and often declines further, especially when the strength of the reward fades or the threat of punishment elapses. This finding suggests that attempts to foster adherence using rewards or punishments are likely to be effective only in the very short term. Indeed, as will be discussed later, most studies of adherence-promoting interventions show just this pattern, of initial benefit with poor maintenance of gains over time (Cortina et al. 2013).

On the other hand, providing people with choices tends to enhance intrinsic motivation (Deci and Ryan 2000). As Deci and Ryan (2008) note, "when people are rewarded, threatened, surveilled, or evaluated, they tend to feel pressured and controlled," whereas being given the opportunity to make choices enhances their sense of behaving autonomously (Deci and Ryan 1987). People resist being controlled and are unlikely to continue a behavior they feel they are being forced to do.

The critical factor here is *autonomy*, which is seen as one of three core psychological needs (the other two being *competence* and *relatedness*). Autonomy refers to "acting with a sense of volition and the experience of willingness" (Deci and Ryan 2012), that your actions are based on your own values, goals, and desires. The opposite of behaving autonomously is being controlled. Extrinsic motivators (rewards) are often effective in helping people *initiate* a behavior change, but their effect rarely lasts. *Maintaining* a behavior change requires that the motivation be internalized, to become the person's own; and internalization depends on the person's belief that she is acting on her own volition and is capable of doing what needs to be done (Ryan et al. 2008).

The concept of autonomy as understood within SDT potentially provides a way of understanding the ways in which the goals of different actors (child, parent, healthcare provider) interact to promote or impede adherence. The theory would predict that approaches taken by parents and providers that make the child feel controlled or coerced would backfire, resulting in poorer adherence, whereas approaches that are autonomy-supportive would result in better adherence over time. There is certainly strong though indirect evidence to support this prediction with regards to teens, as will be discussed in Chaps. 6 and 10.

Numerous studies have validated the importance of autonomy for adult health-behaviors. In one study of adults, having a sense of autonomy (as reflected in questionnaire items such as "Improving my health is something that I am doing by my own choice") accounted for 68 % of the variance in self-report of medication adherence and pill counts (Williams et al. 1998). Autonomy and autonomy-supportive clinician practices have also been shown to relate to improvement in glycemic control in adults with type 2 diabetes (Williams et al. 2004; Williams et al. 2009).

Fewer studies have explicitly examined the importance of sense of autonomy in pediatric adherence. In an observational study of children aged 2–8 years with type 1 diabetes and their mothers, Chisholm et al. (2011) found that children whose mothers involved their children in decision-making during a diabetes-related problem-solving task and used "gentle guidance" (e.g., suggestions) rather than commands had better adherence to dietary restrictions and showed a trend for better glycemic control. They concluded that "treatment adherence and health are optimized when children are offered developmentally sensitive opportunities to participate in decisions about their diabetes care," and that "maternal statements which are 'autonomy supportive' and which promote shared responsibility are key features of children's treatment cooperation." Gillison et al. (2006) found associations between intrinsic (versus extrinsic) motivators and perceived self-determination, and between self-determination and exercise behaviors in over 500 adolescents in the UK. In an older study of youth with type 1 diabetes, Karoly and Bay (1990) found worse metabolic control when youth felt that disease-management goals amounted to being "told what to do" by their parents, versus goals that were self-selected.

More indirect support for the importance of autonomy comes from the general parenting literature, which has consistently shown a strong relation between *authoritative parenting*—that is, parenting that involves high levels of limit-setting in combination with warmth and autonomy support—and health outcomes in a range of areas (see Chap. 7).

Finally, it has recently been recognized that there is substantial overlap, conceptually and practically, between SDT and motivational interviewing (MI)(Patrick and Williams 2012). MI is a clinical approach to fostering behavior change by aligning with the patient, helping the patient explore ambivalence to change, and supporting change that is congruent with the patient's goals and values. MI originally evolved out of clinical experience and has largely been atheoretical, and it has been suggested that SDT might provide the theoretical background for understanding how and why MI works (Markland et al. 2005). MI has a growing evidence-base for adherence promotion in teens, as discussed in Chap. 4.

Autonomy versus independence Finally, it is important to note a distinction made in SDT between *autonomy* and *independence* (Deci and Ryan 2012). As noted earlier, autonomy means acting out of a sense of willingness and volition—doing what *you* want to do. In contrast, independence means acting by yourself, on your own. Logically, these are separate concepts. One can willingly decide to be independent or to be dependent, i.e. whether or not to rely on someone else. In other words, the opposite of autonomy is not dependence, but heteronomy, or lack of volition—i.e., being (or feeling) controlled (Soenens et al. 2007). Thus, SDT identifies two

Fig. 2.2 Dimensions of
autonomy/heteronomy and
dependence/independence

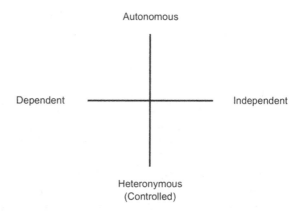

orthogonal dimensions: autonomy/heteronomy (i.e., being controlled) and dependence/independence (Fig. 2.2).

For example, patients may autonomously accept being dependent upon the knowledge and expertise of healthcare providers—in fact, explicit directions are often exactly what people go to professionals for (Patrick and Williams 2012), and this is especially likely to be so in emergency situations where quick decisions must be made. Similarly, youth may autonomously choose to rely on their parents to make decisions for them in certain situations where they feel they lack the competence or maturity—again, medical decision-making is an obvious example. Pushing people to make independent choices in these situations, when they are asking for help, is likely to prove frustrating and counter-productive. In fact, as we will argue later (Chap. 10), pushing independence prematurely is a major contributor to problematic adherence and poor illness control, whereas sharing responsibility while supporting patient autonomy is more likely to ensure better adherence while still promoting adolescent development.

Competence and Relatedness The other two core needs according to SDT are *competence* and *relatedness*. Competence in SDT appears to be very similar in concept to self-efficacy (Bandura 1997), which as noted earlier has a primary place in most (adult) models of adherence. Relatedness in SDT is the sense of being connected to others, and it has been suggested that people are more likely to adopt behaviors "promoted by those to whom they feel connected and in whom they trust" (Ryan et al. 2008). A large body of evidence indicates that parental warmth and parent-child closeness are related to better adherence; there is also evidence that a trusting patient-provider relationship also fosters improved adherence, at least in adults. We will return to these issues in Chaps. 7 and 11.

Putting It All Together

In this chapter we have reviewed a number of prominent theories of adherence viewed through the lens of family-management. The main points are outlined below:

- A child's chronic illness is a stressor to which the child and family must adapt
- Adaptation is a function of child and parent coping, family teamwork, and risk and protective factors.
- Secondary (accommodative) coping is associated with better psychosocial adjustment, but in some circumstances may impede optimal adherence
- Adjustment to illness also involves coming to an understanding of what the illness means to the patient and his/her family
- Child and parent beliefs about the illness, its treatment, their healthcare providers, and their own capabilities influence their goals and how they go about managing the illness
- When children, parents, and/or healthcare providers have different beliefs or goals, conflict can result and management suffers
- Effective goal-setting therefore requires coordination between children, their parents, and their healthcare providers
- Pursing a goal requires self-regulation, or controlling competing impulses that may provide some short-term gain but are contrary to attainment of the goal
- Goals that reflect intrinsic motivations are more likely to be "owned" by the child and maintained over time
- The ways in which parents and healthcare providers try to foster adherence strongly affect the child's success or failure
  - When the child feels coerced or controlled, adherence is likely to suffer
  - When the child feels supported in making choices for him/herself, adherence is likely to be better
  - Supporting a child's autonomy (promoting choice) does not mean pressuring a child to become more independent—autonomy and independence are distinct.

A preliminary conclusion at this stage is that communication and coordination between children, their parents, and their healthcare providers is likely critical to align goals and minimize conflict around chronic illness management. A second major point, which has been touched on in this chapter and for which we will examine the evidence in Chap. 11, is that autonomy support is generally associated with better child adherence, whereas greater child independence is associated with worse adherence and worse illness control. Putting these two ideas together yields the overarching theme of this book, that optimal illness management will be attained when the "triadic partnership" of child, parent, and provider (De Civita and Dobkin 2004) work together.

References

Abrams MA, Klass P, Dreyer BP. Health literacy and children: introduction. Pediatrics 2009;124:262–4 (DeWalt and Hink, Pediatrics 2009;124;265).
Adams CD, Dreyer ML, Dinakar C, Portnoy JM. Pediatric asthma: a look at adherence from the patient and family perspective. Curr Allergy Asthma Rep. 2004;4(6):425–32.

Ajzen I. The theory of planned behavior. Org Behav Hum Decis Process. 1991;50: 179–211.

Ajzen I. The social psychology of decision making. In Higgins ET, Kruglanski AW, Editors. Social psychology: handbook of basic principles. New York: Guilford; 1996. pp. 297–328.

Ajzen I. Theory of planned behavior. http://www-unix.oit.umass.edu/~aizen/tpb.html (2005) Accessed 12 May 2005.

Bandura A. Self-efficacy: The exercise of control. New York: Freeman 1997.

Baumeister RF, Bratslavsky E, Muraven M, Tice DM. Ego depletion: Is the active self a limited resource? Journal of Personality and Social Psychology. 1998;74:1252–65.

Bond GG., Aiken LS., Somerville SC. The health belief model and adolescents with insulin-dependent diabetes mellitus. Health Psychol. 1992;11:190–8.

Bush and Iannotti. A Children's Health Belief Model. Med Care 1990;28:69–86.

Buston KM, Wood SF. Non-compliance amongst adolescents with asthma: listening to what they tell us about self-management. Fam Pract. 2000;17(2):134–8.

Cameron FJ, Northam EA, Ambler G, Daneman D. Routine psychological screening in youth with type 1 diabetes and their parents: a notion whose time has come? Diabetes Care. 2007;30:2716–24.

Charron-Prochownik D, Becker M, Brown M, Liang W, Bennett S. Understanding young children's health benefits and diabetes regimen adherence. Diabetes Educ. 1993;19;409–18.

Chisholm V, Atkinson L, Donaldson C, Noyes K, Payne A, Kelnar C. Maternal communication style, problem-solving and dietary adherence in young children with type 1 diabetes. Clin Child Psychol Psychiatry. 2011;16(3):443–58.

Cline VD, Schwartz DD, Axelrad ME, Anderson BJ. A pilot study of acute stress symptoms in parents and youth following diagnosis of type 1 diabetes. J Clin Psychol Med Settings. 2011;18:416–22.

Compas BE, Jaser SS, Dunn MJ, Rodriguez EM. Coping with chronic illness in childhood and adolescence. Annu Rev Clin Psychol 2012;8:455–80.

Cortina S, Somers M, Rohan JM, Drotar D. Clinical effectiveness of comprehensive psychological intervention for nonadherence to medical treatment: a case series. J Pediatr Psychol. 2013;38:649–63.

De Civita M, Dobkin PL. Pediatric adherence as a multidimensional and dynamic construct, involving a triadic partnership. J Ped Psychol. 2004;29:157–69.

De Ridder DT, De Wit JB. Self-regulation in health behavior: Concepts, theories, and central issues. Self-Regul Health Behav. 2006;1–23.

Deci EL, Ryan RM. The support of autonomy and the control of behavior. Journal of Personality and Social Psychology 1987;53:1024–37.

Deci EL, Ryan RM. The "what" and "why" of goal pursuits: Human needs and the self-determination of behavior. Psychol Inq. 2000;11:227–68.

Deci EL, Ryan RM. Facilitating optimal motivation and psychological well-being across life's domains. Can Psychol. 2008;49:14–23.

Deci EL, Ryan RM. Self-determination theory in health care and its relations to motivational interviewing: a few comments. Int J Behav Nutr Phys Act. 2012;9:24.

Deci EL, Koestner R, Ryan RM. A meta-analytic review of experiments examining the effects of extrinsic rewards on intrinsic motivation. Psych Bull. 1999;125:627–88.

De Walt DA, Hink A. Health literacy and child health outcomes: a systematic review of the literature. Pediatrics 2009;124:265–74.

Diekema DS. Improving childhood vaccination rates. Engl J Med. 2012;366:391–3.

DiMatteo MR. Practitioner-family-patient communication in pediatric adherence: Implications for research and clinical practice. In Drotar D, Editor. Promoting adherence to medical treatment in chronic childhood chronic illness: concepts, methods, and interventions. Mahwah: Erlbaum; 2000. pp. 237–58.

Epstein RM, Street RL. The values and value of patient-centered care. Ann Fam Med 2011;9:100–3.

Funnell MM. Helping patients take charge of their chronic illnesses. Fam Pract Manage 2000 Mar;7(3):47–51.

Gelman SA, Legare CH. Concepts and folk theories. Ann. Rev. Anthropol 2011;40:379–98.

Gibbons FX. Intention, expectation, and willingness 2008. http://cancercontrol.cancer.gov/BRP/constructs/intent-expect-willingness/iew4.html.

Gillison FB, Standage M, Skevington SM. Relationships among adolescents' weight perceptions, exercise goals, exercise motivation, quality of life and leisure-time exercise behaviour: a self-determination theory approach. Health Educ Res. 2006;21(6):836–47.

Graves MM, Roberts MC, Rapoff M, Boyer A. The efficacy of adherence interventions for chronically ill children: a meta-analytic review. J Pediatr Psychol. 2010;35:368–82.

Grey M, Berry D. Coping skills training and problem solving in diabetes. Curr Diab Rep. 2004 Apr;4(2):126–31.

Haller D, Sanci Lena, Sawyer S, et al. Do young people's illness beliefs affect health care? A systematic view. J Adolescent Health 2008;42:436–49.

Helman CG. Disease versus illness in general practice. J Royal Coll Gen Pract. 1981;31:548–52.

Herge WM, Streisand R, Chen R, Holmes C, Kumar A, Mackey ER. Family and youth factors associated with health beliefs and health outcomes in youth with Type 1 diabetes. J Pediatr Psychol. 2012;37:980–9.

Hood KK, Peterson CM, Rohan JM, Drotar D. Association between adherence and glycemic control in pediatric type 1 diabetes: A meta-analysis. Pediatrics. 2009;124:e1171–79.

Janz NK, Becker MH. The health belief model: a decade later. Health Educ Behav 1984; 11(1):1–47.

Kahana S, Drotar D, Frazier T. Meta-analysis of psychological interventions to promote adherence to treatment in pediatric chronic health conditions. J Pediatr Psychol. 2008;33:590–611.

Karoly P, Bay RC. Diabetes self-care goals and their relation to children's metabolic control. J Pediatr Psychol. 1990:15;83–95.

Kazak AE, Stuber ML, Barakat LP, Meeske K, Guthrie D, Meadows AT. Predicting posttraumatic stress symptoms in mothers and fathers of survivors of childhood cancers. J Am Acad Child Adolesc Psychiatry. 1998;37(8):823–31.

Kelly MC, Jill SH, Kathleen L, Cabana MD. The impact of parents' medication beliefs on asthma management. Pediatrics. 2007;120;e521. doi: 10.1542/peds.2006–3023

La Greca AM, Bearman KJ. If an apple a day keeps the doctor away, why is adherence so hard? J Pediatr Psychol. 2001;26:279–82.

La Greca AM, Mackey ER. Adherence to pediatric treatment regimens. In Roberts MC, Steele RG, Editors. Handbook of pediatric psychology. 4th Edn. NY: Guilford; 2009.

Landolt MA, Ribi K, Laimbacher J, Vollrath M, Gnehm HE, Sennhauser FH. Brief report: Posttraumatic stress disorder in parents of children with newly diagnosed type 1 diabetes. J Pediatr Psychol. 2002:27(7):647–52.

Markland D, Ryan RM, Tobin VJ, Rollnick, S. Motivational interviewing and self-determination Theory. J Soc Clin Psychol. 2005;24:811–31.

Marteau TM, Johnston M, Baum JD, Bloch S. Goals of treatment in diabetes: a comparison of doctors and parents of children with diabetes. J Behav Med.1987;10:33–48.

McClure SM, Laibson DI, Lowenstein G, Cohen JD. Separate neural systems value immediate and delayed monetary rewards. Science. 2004;306:503–7.

Metcalfe J, Mischel W. A hot/cool-system analysis of delay of gratification: dynamics of willpower. Psychol Rev. 1999;106:3–19.

Mischel W, Ayduk O. Willpower in a cognitive-affective processing system: The dynamics of delay of gratification. In Baumeister RF, Vohs KD, Editors, Handbook of self-regulation: research, theory, and applications. New York: Guilford; 2004. pp. 99–129.

Naar-King S. Arfken C. Frey M. Harris M. Secord E. Ellis D. Psychosocial factors and treatment adherence in paediatric HIV/AIDS. AIDS Care. 2006;18:621–8.

Patino AM, Sanchez J, Eidson M, Delamater AM. Health beliefs and regimen adherence in minority adolescents with type 1 diabetes. J pediatr psychol. 2005;30(6):503–12.

Patrick H, Williams GC. Self-determination theory: its application to health behavior and complementarity with Motivational Interviewing. Int J Beh Nutr Phys Act. 2012;9:18.

Rapoff MA. Adherence to pediatric medical regimens. 2nd ed. New York: Springer; 2010.

Rehm RS, Franck LS. Long-term goals and normalization strategies of children and families affected by HIV/AIDS. Adv Nurs Sci. 2000;23:69–82.

Reid GJ, Dubow EF, Carey TC, Dura JR. Contribution of coping to medical adjustment and treatment responsibility among children and adolescents with diabetes. J Dev Beh Ped. 1994;15:327–35.

Rich M, Patashnick J, Chalfen R. Visual illness narratives of asthma: explanatory models and health-related behavior. Am J Health Behav 2002;26(6):442–53.

Riekert KA, Drotar D. The beliefs about medication scale: development, reliability, and validity. J Clin Psychol Med. 2002;9(2):177–84.

Rudolph KD, Dennig MD, Weisz JR. Determinants and consequences of children's coping in the medical setting: conceptualization, review, and critique. Psych Bull. 1995;118(3):328.

Ryan RM, Deci EL. Self-determination theory and the facilitation of intrinsic motivation, social development, and well-being. Ame Psychol. 2000;55:68.

Ryan RM, Patrick H, Deci EL, Williams GC. Facilitating health behaviour change and its maintenance: Interventions based on self-determination theory. Eur Health Psychol. 2008;10:2–5.

Sameroff A, Editor. The transactional model of development: how children and contexts shape each other. Washington, DC: American Psychological Association; 2009.

Schwartz L, Drotar D. Defining the nature and impact of goals in children and adolescents with a chronic health condition: A review of research and a theoretical framework. J Clin Psychol Med Settings. 2006;13:393–405.

Skinner TC, Hampson SE. Social support and personal models of diabetes in relation to self-care and well-being in adolescents with type 1 diabetes mellitus. J Adolesc. 1998;21:703–15.

Skinner TC, Hampson SE. Personal models of diabetes in relation to self-care and well-being, and glycemic control. A prospective study in adolescence. Diabetes Care. 2001;24:828–33.

Skinner CT, Hampson SE, Fife-Schaw CR. Personality, personal model beliefs, and self-care in adolescents and young adults with Type 1 diabetes. Health Psychol. 2002;21(1):61–70.

Soenens B, Vansteenkiste M, Lens W, Luyckx K, Goossens L, Beyers W, Ryan RM. Conceptualizing parental autonomy support: Adolescent perceptions of promotion of independence versus promotion of volitional functioning. Dev Psychol. 2007;43:633–46.

Strecher VJ, Rosenstock IM. The health belief model. In: Glantz K, Lewis FM, Rimer BK, Editors. Health behavior and health education: theory, research, and practice. 2nd edn. San Francisco: Jossey-Bass; 1997. pp. 41–59.

Thompson RJ Jr, Gustafson KE. Adaptation to chronic childhood illness. Washington, DC: American Psychological Association; 1996.

Turner T, Cull WL, Bayldon B, et al. Pediatricians and health literacy: descriptive results from a national survey. Pediatrics.2009;124(5 suppl):S299–305.

Urquhart Law G, Kelly TP, Huey D, et al. Self-management and well-being in adolescents with diabetes mellitus: do illness representations play a regulatory role? J Adolesc Health 2002;31(4):381–85.

US Department of Health and Human Services. Healthy people 2010. Washington, DC: US Government Printing Office; 2000.

Wade S, Weil C, Holden G, et al. Psychosocial characteristics of inner-city children with asthma: a description of the NCICAS psychosocial protocol. Pediatr Pulmonol. 1997;24(4):263–276.

Wallander JL, Varni JW. Effects of pediatric chronic physical disorders on child and family adjustment. J Child Psychol Psychiatry 1998;39:29–46.

Williams GC. Improving patients' health through supporting the autonomy of patients and providers. In Deci EL, Ryan RM, Editors. Handbook of self-determination research. Rochester: University of Rochester Press; 2002. pp. 233–54.

Williams GC, Freedman ZR, Deci EL. Supporting autonomy to motivate patients with diabetes for glucose control. Diabetes Care. 1998;21:1644–51.

Williams GC, McGregor HA, Zeldman A, Freedman ZR, Deci EL. Testing a self-determination theory process model for promoting glycemic control through diabetes self-management. Health Psychol. 2004;23:58–66.

Williams GC, Heather P, Christopher P Niemiec L. Keoki W, George D, Lafata JE, Heisler M, Tunceli K, Pladevall M. Reducing the health risks of diabetes how self-determination theory may help improve medication adherence and quality of life. Diabetes Educ. 2009;35(3):484–92.

Wilson RA, Kei FC, Editors. The MIT encyclopedia of the cognitive sciences. Massachusetts: MIT; 2001.

Wolfe J, Klar N, Grier HE, Duncan J, Salem-Schatz S, Emanuel EJ, et al. Understanding of prognosis among parents of children who died of cancer. JAMA. 2000;284:2469–75.

Yin HS, Johnson M, Mendelsohn AL, Abrams MA, Sanders LM, Dreyer BP. The health literacy of parents in the United States: a nationally representative study. Pediatrics. 2009;124(5 suppl):S289–98.

Zebracki K, Drotar D. Outcome expectancy and self-efficacy in adolescent asthma self-management. Child Health Care. 2004;33(2):133–49.

Chapter 3
Barriers and Facilitators of Adherence

Marisa E. Hilliard

Abstract Contributors to a person's adherence or non-adherence are complex, varied, and highly individual. Yet common themes have emerged and show that barriers to and facilitators of adherence occur on multiple levels: individual, family, healthcare systems, and cultural issues. Some predictors of adherence are stable or fixed and must be considered in clinical care delivery, research, and policy, while other contributors have the potential to be modified through targeted clinical intervention strategies. This chapter will review predictors of adherence in youth with chronic conditions across these multiple levels.

Clinical Factors

There is mixed evidence regarding the impact of specific disease or treatment characteristics on an individual's treatment adherence. For example, greater disease severity (e.g., number of symptoms or comorbidities) or higher complexity of a treatment regimen (e.g., time demands of treatments, number of medications) have been inconsistently linked with adherence rates in adult and pediatric populations (Bugni et al. 2012, Eakin et al. 2011, Ingersoll and Cohen 2008, Lindsay and Heaney 2013, Sherman et al. 2001). While some data demonstrate lower adherence rates among more complex diseases or regimens, other data indicate no relationship. An important distinction is that while objective rankings of severity and complexity may or may not be related to adherence, an individual's *perception* of greater disease severity or treatment complexity shows a more consistent relation with poorer adherence (Chandwani et al. 2012; DiMatteo et al. 2007; Reed-Knight et al. 2011). That is, patients who perceive their own disease to be more severe or complex are less likely to adhere to prescribed treatments than patients who view their condition as milder or easier to manage.

Similarly, some data suggest that adherence worsens with longer disease duration (Reed-Knight et al. 2011; Hilliard et al. 2013), although this is not evident in

M. E. Hilliard (✉)
Department of Pediatrics, Section of Psychology,
Baylor College of Medicine, Houston, Texas, USA
e-mail: marisa.hilliard@bcm.edu

© Springer International Publishing Switzerland 2015
D. D. Schwartz, M. E. Axelrad, *Healthcare Partnerships for Pediatric Adherence,*
SpringerBriefs in Public Health, DOI 10.1007/978-3-319-13668-4_3

other studies (Eakin et al. 2011). With longer disease duration, the unrelenting demands of disease management may accumulate and lead to greater disease burnout or distress. On the other hand, longer disease duration may provide more opportunity for individuals to identify useful coping strategies and develop a sense of mastery over their treatments. It is possible that experiences such as these that emerge with longer disease duration may have a stronger, more direct association with changes in adherence behaviors than disease duration itself.

Together, results suggest that adherence is linked to an individual's subjective experience of having and managing a complex chronic condition more than objective clinical characteristics, such as severity, complexity, or duration.

Individual factors

Although patterns of adherence are highly individual and are impacted by numerous factors and experiences, trends have emerged with relation to personal characteristics. For example, older youth age is generally linked with lower adherence (Hilliard et al. 2013; Kahana et al. 2008; McQuaid et al. 2003; Pai and Ostenorf 2011; Williams et al. 2006), although the association is not always evident (Sherman et al. 2001). Decreasing adherence at older youth ages likely reflects developmental changes that occur during adolescence, such as shifts in self-management responsibility from parents to youth and faster increases in desire for autonomy compared with self-management skills (see Chap. 10). Cognitive development (e.g., executive functioning, working memory, organization, behavioral planning, problem-solving) improves across childhood and into adolescence and can facilitate better adherence (McNally et al. 2010; O'Hara and Holmbeck 2013), yet this growth may not match the level of self-management autonomy expected of adolescents with chronic conditions (Wysocki et al. 1996). Combined, normative developmental shifts can often result in a net deficit for an individual's capacity to consistently and accurately adhere to a complex treatment regimen.

Chronic Illness and Mental Health Children with a chronic illness are at elevated risk for psychosocial and mental health concerns (Drotar 2006). Most adapt well and experience similar quality of life as their peers, but a substantial minority experience symptoms of distress that reach clinical levels, and these children tend to have poorer health outcomes and quality of life. For some, the diagnosis of a chronic medical illness is a traumatic event that can be associated with symptoms of post traumatic stress. Approximately one in six children will experience symptoms of acute stress following a diagnosis of cancer (Kazak et al. 2012) or type 1 diabetes (Cline et al. 2011). Rates may even be higher in pediatric transplant patients (Shemesh et al. 2000). One in three children will meet criteria for an adjustment disorder at diagnosis, and these children are at heightened risk for long term problems with depression and anxiety (e.g., Grey et al. 1995). For others, living with a chronic illness becomes a chronic stressor over time, precipitating the onset of mental health concerns like depression or anxiety, or exacerbating pre-existing problems. For example, youth with type 1 diabetes have rates of depressive symptoms approximately twice as high as in the general population (Hood et al. 2006).

Mental health concerns can have a dramatic negative impact on adherence and illness control. Depression, as well as subclinical symptoms of depression and distress, are of particular concern (Gray et al. 2012; Hilliard et al. 2013; Kahana et al. 2008; McGrady and Hood 2010; Pai and Ostenorf 2011; Garvie et al. 2011). Depressive symptoms include difficulties with the initiation, motivation, and follow-through necessary for engaging in self-care behaviors (Gonzalez et al. 2008; McGrady et al. 2009; McGrady and Hood 2010). Depressive symptoms can also color one's beliefs about the importance of treatments or motivation to adhere to prescribed regimens (Hilliard et al. 2014). Although infrequent youth with suicidal ideation are more than three times more likely to be nonadherent to a medical regimen (Goldston et al. 1997).

Disordered eating behaviors have also been shown to be negatively associated with adherence. Youth with diabetes and disordered eating behaviors may intentionally omit taking their insulin as a strategy to control their weight, placing them at high risk for DKA (Goebel-Fabbri et al. 2008).

Post-traumatic stress (PTS) is also associated with much poorer adherence and illness control. For example, for children who have received a solid organ transplant and have transplant-related PTS or PTSD, taking immunosuppressant medication may act as a reminder of the transplant and may lead to significant avoidance of disease-management tasks, making transplant failure much more likely (Shemesh 2004; Shemesh et al. 2000).

Finally, disease-related distress and negative emotional experiences and affect around recommended medications and treatments are also linked with health behaviors and outcomes (Hilliard et al. 2013; Maikranz et al. 2007). For instance, experiencing disease burnout or feeling frustrated by difficult-to-control disease symptoms may make it more difficult for youth to adhere to demanding treatment regimens.

Externalizing behavior problems are also associated with suboptimal adherence (Cohen et al. 2004; Gerson et al. 2004; Holmes et al. 2006; Northam et al. 2005). Children with chronic illness and comorbid behavior problems may be at especially high risk for problems with regimen adherence and illness control, as they are more likely to resist complying with parent or provider requests to participate in management tasks.

Positive Characteristics In contrast to the negative impact of psychological concerns on adherence, positive personal characteristics and experiences are associated with optimal disease management. Optimism and hope, for instance, have demonstrated some associations with adherence and disease control (Maikranz et al. 2007; Lloyd et al. 2009). Experiencing high levels of social support have also been shown to promote youths' engagement with disease self-management behaviors in some studies (MacDonnell et al. 2010, Naar-King et al. 2013), although not all findings support this conclusion (Palladino and Helgeson 2012).

Health Beliefs Finally, individual perspectives about one's diagnosis and prescribed treatment may influence one's health-related behaviors. Although less well-studied in youth as compared to adults, evidence is emerging that young people's adherence may be influenced by their personal health beliefs regarding the perceived necessity or helpfulness of their prescribed treatments (Bucks et al. 2009; Feldman et al., 2007). Health beliefs related to adherence include the degree to which an individual perceives his/her disease as a threat (DiMatteo et al. 2007; Garvie et al. 2011), one's readiness or motivation to begin engaging in behaviors to manage the disease (MacDonell et al. 2010), and one's sense of confidence or self-efficacy in their ability to execute the tasks of self-management (Ott et al. 2000).

In some diseases, perceptions about the necessity or importance of treatment may be impacted by knowledge of or about one's diagnosis or condition. For example, among youth with prenatally acquired HIV, the diagnosis has been disclosed to some children and not to others. Youths' awareness of their positive HIV status has been associated with better adherence to daily antiretroviral medications (Bikaako-Kajura et al. 2006). However, this finding is not consistent (Williams et al. 2006), and in other chronic conditions for which diagnosis disclosure to the child is not as prominent an issue (e.g., asthma, Ho et al. 2003; sickle cell disease, Jensen et al. 2005) neither child nor caregiver knowledge about the disease and its potential consequences show a reliable relation with adherence. Low health literacy may be important to adherence as it may limit one's knowledge about and understanding of their disease, and this can impact engagement in health behaviors such as medication adherence (DeWalt and Hink 2009)

Family Factors

Various aspects of family relationships have been investigated in relation to youths' adherence to medical treatments. One of the most thoroughly evidenced conclusions about family disease management across conditions is that negative parent-child relationships, often characterized by elevated levels of family conflict, are linked with suboptimal adherence and health outcomes (Hilliard et al. 2013, De Lambo et al. 2004; Gerson et al. 2004; Naar-King et al. 2013; Reed-Knight et al. 2011).

One hypothesized mechanism linking poor relationships and conflict with suboptimal adherence is that conflictive or unsupportive family interactions may reduce youth's self-efficacy and ultimately deter engagement in adherence behaviors (Ott et al. 2000). It is plausible that youth would wish to avoid situations that cause conflict, such as those related to disease management. Conflict may also interfere with family communication and problem-solving related to disease-management tasks.

On the other hand, positive aspects of family relationships are also associated with adherence, such as parental acceptance (O'Hara and Holmbeck 2013), openness and supportive interactions (Butow et al. 2010), and family cohesion (Mackey et al. 2011). Many of these positive aspects of the parent-child relationship are captured within the authoritative parenting style, which is characterized as providing firm and consistent structure yet loving and warm interactions, and has been associated with better adherence (Monaghan et al. 2012; see Chap. 7). Families who interact in positive ways may have more effective communication, more successfully encourage youth to engage in adherence behaviors, and provide more reinforcement for successfully completing adherence tasks (DiMatteo 2004). Communication and problem-solving among family members regarding expectations for adherence may also be more successful in families characterized by cooperative and cohesive interactions.

Given the potential mismatch between the complex demands of chronic condition management and youths' developing autonomy and cognitive abilities, parents and family members are integral to the completion of daily disease management tasks. Indeed, the degree to which parents and family members are actively involved in youths' disease management is consistently associated with treatment adherence; more consistent, collaborative involvement is associated with better adherence to treatments for numerous pediatric chronic conditions (Reed-Knight et al. 2011; Wysocki et al. 2009), while children having primary or sole responsibility for self-management is a well-documented risk factor (Kahana et al. 2008; Chap. 10). For younger children or those with self-management limitations, developmentally appropriate involvement includes parents or caregivers completing disease management tasks, while for older or more autonomous youth, consistent parental monitoring of youths' own adherence to disease management tasks is beneficial (Modi et al. 2008; Ellis et al. 2007). One component of this association is the facilitation of effective communication and teamwork around disease management. For example, family members who agree about the distribution of responsibility among one another tend to demonstrate better adherence (Martin et al. 2007).

Parents' stress and psychological functioning play important roles in their ability to support children's adherence to medical regimens. Many parents of youth with chronic conditions report elevated levels of parenting stress, which has been associated with more difficulty with adherence (DeMore et al. 2005; Gerson et al. 2004; Mitchell et al. 2009; Monaghan et al. 2012). Elevated levels of parental (especially maternal) symptoms of clinical distress, including posttraumatic stress or depressive symptoms, have also been linked with poorer youth adherence (Bartlett et al. 2004; Horsch and McManus 2013; Streisand et al. 2008).

Healthcare System and Provider Factors

The associations between healthcare system characteristics and adherence have primarily been studied in adult health settings, and less is currently known with relation to pediatric adherence. Healthcare providers' communication skills and interpersonal style have been a focus of previous research. Among adults, patient perceptions of providers displaying empathy, asking questions, building rapport, and addressing both medical *and* psychosocial issues during medical visits represent good communication, and more than double the likelihood of optimal adherence (Zolnierek and DiMatteo 2009). The importance of good patient-family-provider communication in pediatrics has also been emphasized, particularly in relation to education about medications and in building a trusting relationship (DiMatteo 2004).

Related to the patient-provider relationship is the concept of "white coat compliance [adherence]," a term that represents patients' increase in adherence immediately prior to a medical visit (Dusing et al. 2001). This pattern has been demonstrated for antiepileptic medication adherence in youth with epilepsy (Modi et al. 2012) and for blood glucose monitoring in youth with type 1 diabetes (Driscoll et al. 2011), suggesting that some anticipation about the upcoming clinic visit may be impacting youths' adherence across diseases.

Cultural and Socioeconomic Factors

Disparities in adherence and health outcomes across racial, ethnic, and socioeconomic groups are a widespread and well-documented problem in pediatrics (Gallegos-Macias et al. 2003; Jarzembowski et al. 2004; Naar-King et al. 2013; McQuaid et al. 2003; Powell et al. 2013). Youth from racial and ethnic minority groups tend to demonstrate poorer adherence to recommended treatments in a number of chronic conditions. These disparities are likely attributable to multiple factors (Chap. 9), including barriers that are disproportionately experienced by minority youth and families such as more limited access to quality healthcare, poorer insurance coverage, and fewer socioeconomic resources (Mayberry et al. 2000; Pai and Ostenorf 2011; Powell et al. 2013).

There is also evidence that health care providers themselves tend to be less adherent to care guidelines in treating youth from minority and underserved populations (Ortega et al. 2002) and use less positive communication styles (Johnson et al. 2004). Such differences in some pediatricians' care of minority patients may be explained in part by implicit biases (Sabin and Greenwald 2012) and have the potential to impact adherence and ultimately contribute to health disparities.

Summary

Multiple factors help or hinder adherence in pediatric populations, including patient characteristics, parent and family functioning, and healthcare system factors. Moreover, these factors interact in complex ways that we are only beginning to unravel. Interactions between children and parents and between families and healthcare providers are important contributors to child health outcomes, and are themselves influenced by broader socio-cultural factors. Table 3.1 summarizes key barriers and facilitators of adherence in each domain. In the next chapter we review evidence-based interventions targeted at these different factors.

Table 3.1 Multi-level barriers and facilitators of adherence to pediatric regimens

Level	Barriers	Facilitators
Individual	Older age Increasing self-management responsibilities may not match abilities Depressive symptoms, disease-related distress, burnout Low health literacy	Optimism, hopefulness Self-efficacy for self-management Social support High motivation, readiness, and perceived importance of adherence
Family	Conflict about disease or regimen Caregivers over- or under-involved in daily disease management Miscarried helping Disagreement in family roles or responsibilities for disease management Parental stress or psychological symptoms	Collaborative parent involvement in disease management Effective problem-solving as a family Open, supportive family communication style Parental support of youth self-management Family cohesion Authoritative parenting style
Systems	Racial/ethnic disparities in health care access and health outcomes Limited financial resources, insurance	Provider uses empathic communication style, asks questions Provider addresses psychosocial concerns Building trust

References

Bartlett SJ, Krishnan JA, Riekert KA, et al. Maternal depressive symptoms and adherence to therapy in inner-city children with asthma. Pediatr. 2004;113:229–37.

Bikaako-Kajura W, Luyirika E, Purcell DW, et al. Disclosure of HIV status and adherence to daily drug regimens among HIV-infected children in Uganda. AIDS Behav. 2006;10:85–93.

Bucks RS, Hawkins K, Skinner TC, Horn S, Seddon P, Horne R. Adherence to treatment in adolescents with cystic fibrosis: the role of illness perceptions and treatment beliefs. J Pediatr Psychol. 2009;34:893–902.

Bugni VM, Ozaki LS, Okamoto KY, et al. Factors associated with adherence to treatment in children and adolescents with chronic rheumatic diseases. J Pediatr (Rio J). 2012;88:483–8.

Butow P, Palmer S, Pai A, et al. Review of adherence-related issues in adolescents and young adults with cancer. J Clin Oncol. 2010;28:4800–9.

Chandwani S, Loenig LJ, Sill AM, Abramowitz S, Conner LC, D'Angelo L. Predictors of antiretroviral medication adherence among a diverse cohort of adolescents with HIV. J Adolesc Health. 2012;51:242–51.

Cline VD, Schwartz DD, Axelrad ME, Anderson BJ. A pilot study of acute stress symptoms in parents and youth following diagnosis of type I diabetes. J Clin Psychol Med Settings. 2011;18:416–22.

Cohen DM, Lumley MA, Naar-King S, Partridge T, Cakan N. Child behavior problems and family functioning as predictors of adherence and glycemic control in economically disadvantaged children with Type 1 Diabetes: a prospective study. J Pediatr Psychol. 2004;29:171–84.

De Lambo KE, Ievers-Landis CE, Drotar D, Quittner AL. Association of observed family relationship quality and problem-solving skills with treatment adherence in older children and adolescents with cystic fibrosis. J Pediatr Psychol. 2004;29:343–53.

DeMore M, Adams C, Wilson N, Hogan MB. Parenting stress, difficult child behavior, and use of routines in relation to adherence in pediatric asthma. Child Health Care. 2005;34:245–59.

DeWalt DA, Hink A. Health literacy and child health outcomes: a systematic review of the litera-ture. Pediatrics. 2009;124:S265–S74.

DiMatteo MR. The role of effective communication with children and their families in fostering adherence to pediatric regimens. Patient Educ Couns. 2004;55:339–44.

DiMatteo MR, Haskard KB, Williams SL. Health beliefs, disease severity, and patient adherence: a meta-analysis. Med Care. 2007;45:521–8.

Driscoll KA, Johnson SB, Tan Y, et al. Does blood glucose monitoring increase prior to clinic visits in children with type 1 diabetes? Diabetes Care. 2011;34:2170–3.

Drotar D Psychological interventions in childhood chronic illness. Washington, DC: American Psychological Association. 2006.

Dusing R, Lottermoser K, Mengden T. Compliance with drug therapy—new answers to an old question. Nephrol Dial Transplant. 2001;16:1317–21.

Eakin MN, Bilderback A, Boyle MP, Mogayzel PJ, Riekert KA. Longitudinal association be-tween medication adherence and lung health in people with cystic fibrosis. J Cyst Fibros. 2011;10:258–64.

Ellis DA, Podolski C, Frey M, et al. The role of parental monitoring in adolescent health outcomes: impact on regimen adherence in youth with type 1 diabetes. J Pediatr Psychol. 2007;32:907–17.

Feldman DE, de Civita M, Dobkin PL, et al. Perceived adherence to prescribed treatment in juve-nile idiopathic arthritis over a one-year period. Arthritis Rheum. 2007;57:226–33.

Gallegos-Macias AR, Macias SR, Kaufman E, Skipper B, Kalishman N. Relationship between glycemic control, ethnicity and socioeconomic status in Hispanic and white non-Hispanic youths with type 1 diabetes mellitus. Pediatr Diabetes. 2003;4:19–23.

Garvie PA, Flynn PM, Belzer M, et al. Psychological factors, beliefs about medication, and adher-ence of youth with human immunodeficiency virus in a multisite directly observed therapy pilot study. J Adol Health. 2011;48:637–40.

Gerson A, Furth S, Neu A, Fivush B. Assessing associations between medication adherence and potentially modifiable psychosocial variables in pediatric kidney transplant recipients and their families. Pediatric Transplantation. 2004;8:543–50.

Goebel-Fabbri AE, Fikkan J, Franko DL, Pearson K, Anderson BJ, Weinger K. Insulin restric-tion and associated morbidity and mortality in women with type 1 diabetes. Diabetes Care. 2008;31:415–9.

Goldston DB, Kelley AE, Reboussin DM, et al. Suicidal ideation and behaviour and noncompli-ance with the medical regimen among diabetic adolescents. J Am Acad Child Adolesc Psychia-try. 1997;36:1528–36.

Gonzalez JS, Peyrot M, McCarl LA, et al. Depression and diabetes treatment non-adherence: a meta-analysis. Diabetes Care. 2008;31:2398–403.

Gray WN, Denson LA, Baldassano RN, Hommel KA. Treatment adherence in adolescents with inflammatory bowel disease: the collective impact of barriers to adherence and anxiety/depres-sive symptoms. J Pediatr Psychol. 2012;37:282–91.

Grey M, Cameron M, Lipman TH, Thurber FW. Psychosocial status of children with diabetes in the first 2 years after diagnosis. Diabetes Care. 1995;18:1330–6.

Hilliard ME, Wu YP, Rausch J, Dolan LM, Hood KK. Predictors of deteriorations in diabetes management and control in adolescents with type 1 diabetes. J Adolesc Health. 2013;52:28–34.

Hilliard ME, Eakin MN, Borrelli B, Green A, Riekert KA. Medication beliefs mediate between de-pressive symptoms and medication adherence in cystic fibrosis. Health Psychol. 2014. Ahead of print: doi:10.1037/hea0000136.

Ho J, Bender BG, Gavin LA, et al. Relations among asthma knowledge, treatment adherence, and outcome. J Allergy Clin Immunol. 2003;111:498–502.

Holmes CS, Chen R, Streisand R, et al. Predictors of youth diabetes care behaviors and metabolic control: a structural equation modeling approach. J Pediatr Psychol. 2006;31:770–84.

Hood KK, Huestis S, Maher A, Butler D, Volkening L, Laffel LM. Depressive symptoms in chil-dren and adolescents with type 1 diabetes: association with diabetes-specific characteristics. Diab Care. 2006;29:1389–91.

Horsch A, McManus F. Maternal posttraumatic stress symptoms are related to adherence to their child's diabetes treatment regimen. J Health Psychol. 2013. doi:10.1177/1359105313482169.

Ingersoll KS, Cohen J. The impact of medication regimen factors on adherence to chronic treatment: a review of literature. J Behav Med. 2008;31:213–24.

Jarzembowski T, John E, Panaro F, et al. Impact of non-compliane on outcome after pediatric kidney transplantation: an analysis in racial subgroups. Pediatr Transplant. 2004;8:367–71.

Jensen SA, Elkin TD, Hilker K, et al. Caregiver knowledge and adherence in children with sickle cell disease: knowing is not doing. J Clin Psychol Med Settings. 2005;12:333–7.

Johnson RL, Roter D, Powe NR, Cooper LA. Patient race/ethnicity and quality of patient-physician communication during medical visits. Am J Public Health. 2004;94:2084–90.

Kahana SY, Frazier TW, Drotar D. Preliminary quantitative investigation of predictors of treatment non-adherence in pediatric transplantation: a brief report. Pediatr Transplant. 2008;12:656–60.

Kazak AE, Brier M, Alderfer MA, Reilly A, Parker SF, Rogerwick S, Ditaranto S, Barakat LP. Screening for psychosocial risk in pediatric cancer. Pediatr Blood Cancer. 2012;59:822–7.

Lindsay JT, Heaney LG. Nonadherence in difficult asthma: facts, myths, and a time to act. Patient Prefer Adherence. 2013;7:329–36.

Lloyd SM, Cantell M, Pacaud D, Crawford S, Dewey D. Hope, perceived maternal empathy, medical regimen adherence, and glycemic control in adolescents with type 1 diabetes. J Pediatr Psychol. 2009;24:1025–9.

MacDonell KE, Naar-King S, Murphy DA, Parsons JT, Harper GW. Predictors of medication adherence in high risk youth of color living with HIV. J Pediatr Psychol. 2010;25:593–601.

Mackey ER, Hilliard ME, Berger SS, et al. Individual and family strengths: an examination of the relation to disease management and metabolic control in youth with type 1 diabetes. Fam Syst Health. 2011;29:314–26.

Maikranz JM, Steele RG, Dreyer ML, Stratman AC, Bovaird JA. The relationship of hope and illness-related uncertainty to emotional adjustment and adherence among pediatric renal and liver transplant recipients. J Pediatr Psychol. 2007;32:571–81.

Martin S, Elliott-DeSorbo DK, Wolters PL, Toledo-Tamula MA, Roby G, Zeichner S, et al. Patient, caregiver and regimen characteristics associated with adherence to highly active antiretroviral therapy among HIV-infected children and adolescents. Pediatr Infect Dis J. 2007;26:61–7.

Mayberry RM, Mili F, Ofili E. Racial and ethnic differences in access to medical care. Med Care Res Rev. 2000;57:108–45.

McGrady ME, Hood KK. Depressive symptoms in adolescents with type 1 diabetes: associations with longitudinal outcomes. Diab Res Clin Pract. 2010;88:e35–e7.

McGrady ME, Laffel L, Drotar D, Repaske D, Hood KK. Depressive symptoms and glycemic control in adolescents with Type 1 Diabetes: mediational role of glucose monitoring. Diabetes Care. 2009;32:804–6.

McNally K, Rohan J, Pendley JS, Delamater A, Drotar D. Executive functioning, treatment adherence, and glycemic control in children with type 1 diabetes. Diabetes Care. 2010;33:1159–62.

McQuaid EL, Kopel SJ, Klein RB, Fritz GK. Medication adherence in pediatric asthma: reasoning, responsibility, and behavior. J Pediatr Psychol. 2003;28:323–33.

Mitchell SJ, Hilliard ME, Mednick L, Henderson C, Logen FR, Streisand R. Stress among fathers of young children with type 1 diabetes. Families, Systems, and Health. 2009;27:314–24.

Modi AC, Marciel KK, Slater SK, Drotar D, Quitter AL. The influence of parental supervision on medical adherence in adolescents with cystic fibrosis: developmental shifts from pre to late adolescence. Child Health Care. 2008;37:78–92.

Modi AC, Ingerski LM, Rausch JR, Glauser TA, Drotar D. White coat adherence over the first year of therapy in pediatric epilepsy. J Pediatr. 2012;161:695–9.

Monaghan M, Horn IB, Alvarez V, Cogen FR, Streisand R. Authoritative parenting, parenting stress, and self-care in pre-adolescents with type 1 diabetes. J Clin Psychol Med Settings. 2012;19:255–61.

Naar-King S, Montepiedra G, Garvie P, Kammerer B, Malee K, Sirois PA, et al. Social ecological predictors of longitudinal HIV treatment adherence in youth with perinatally acquired HIV. J Pediatr Psychol. 2013;38(6):664–74.

Northam EA, Matthews LK, Anderson PJ, Cameron FJ, Werther GA. Psychiatric morbidity and health outcome in Type 1 Diabetes-perspectives from a prospective longitudinal study. Diabet Med. 2005;22:152–7.

O'Hara LK, Holmbeck GN. Executive functions and parenting behaviors in association with medical adherence and autonomy among youth with spina bifida. J Pediatr Psychol. 2013;38:675–87.

Ortega AN, Gergen PJ, Paltiel AD, Bauchner H, Belanger KD, Leaderer BP. Impact of site of care, race, and Hispanic ethnicity on medication use for childhood asthma. Pediatrics. 2002;109:e1–e6.

Ott J, Greening L, Palardy N, Holderby A, DeBell WK. Self-efficacy as a mediator variable for adolescents' adherence to treatment for insulin-dependent diabetes mellitus. Child Healthcare. 2000;29:47–63.

Pai ALH, Ostenorf HM. Treatment adherence in adolescents and young adults affected by chronic illness during the health care transition from pediatric to adult health care: a literature review. Child Health Care. 2011;40:16–33.

Palladino DK, Helgeson VS. Friends or foes? A review of peer influence on self-care and glycemic control in adolescents with type 1 diabetes. J Pediatr Psychol. 2012;37(5):591–603.

Powell PW, Chen R, Kumar A, Streisand R, Holmes CS. Sociodemographic effects on biological, disease care, and diabetes knowledge factors in youth with type 1 diabetes. J Child Health Care. 2013;17:174–85.

Reed-Knight B, Lewis JD, Blount RL. Association of disease, adolescent, and family factors with medication adherence in pediatric inflammatory bowel disease. J Pediatr Psychol. 2011;36:308–17.

Sabin JA, Greenwald AG. The influence of implicit bias on treatment recommendations for 4 common pediatric conditions: pain, urinary tract infection, attention deficit hyperactivity disorder, and asthma. Am J Public Health. 2012;102:988–95.

Shemesh E. Non-adherence to medications following pediatric liver transplantation. Pediatr Transplant. 2004;8:600–5.

Shemesh E, Lurie S, Stuber ML, Emre S, Patel Y, Vohra P, Aromando M, Shneider BL. A pilot study of posttraumatic stress and nonadherence in pediatric liver transplant recipients. Pediatrics. 2000;105:e29–e9.

Sherman J, Patel P, Hutson A, Chesrown S, Hendeles L. Adherence to oral montelukast and inhaled fluticasone in children with persistent asthma. Pharmacotherapy. 2001;21:1464–7.

Streisand R, Mackey ER, Elliot BM, Mednick L, Slaughter IM, Turek J, Austin A. Parental anxiety and depression associated with caring for a child newly diagnosed with type 1 diabetes: opportunities for education and counseling. Patient Education and Counseling. 2008;73:333–8.

Williams PL, Storm D, Montepiedra G, Nichols S, Kammer B, Sirois PA, et al. Predictors of adherence to antiretroviral medications in children and adolescents with HIV infection. Pediatrics. 2006;118:e1745–e57.

Wysocki T, Taylor A, Hough BS, Linscheid TR, Yeates KO, Naglieri JA. Deviation from developmentally appropriate self-care autonomy: association with diabetes outcomes. Diabetes Care. 1996;19(2):119–25.

Wysocki T, Nansel TR, Holmbeck GN, et al. Collaborative involvement of primary and secondary caregivers: associations with youths' diabetes outcomes. J Pediatr Psychol. 2009;34:869–81.

Zolnierek KBH, DiMatteo MR. Physician communication and patient adherence to treatment: a meta-analysis. Med Care. 2009;47:826–34.

Chapter 4
Interventions to Promote Adherence: Innovations in Behavior Change Strategies

Marisa E. Hilliard

Abstract Only in recent years has a large enough body of research on adherence-promoting interventions been amassed so that systematic reviews and meta-analyses of their impact can reliably be evaluated. Overall, these reviews indicate that interventions tend to result in modest improvements in adherence to treatment recommendations and medications, with effect sizes typically in the small to medium range across various chronic condition populations and intervention types. Positive effects on health outcomes have also been reported. This chapter reviews the literature on interventions for pediatric nonadherence, paying special attention to recent innovations that have the potential to expand interventions' reach and effectiveness.

Children and youth identified as struggling with nonadherence often get referred for specialized treatment focused on improving adherence-related behaviors. According to Rapoff (2010), interventions fall under one of several categories:

- *Educational interventions* presume a knowledge deficit on the part of patient or parent and focus on improving knowledge and understanding of the disease, the disease process, and both the rationale and the mechanics of treatment. Educational interventions are often the first line of approach utilized by healthcare providers.
- *Organizational strategies* focus on making the medical regimen more manageable for families, and on making the healthcare system easier to navigate. Examples include simplifying medical regimens, providing organizational tools such as labeled pill boxes, recording logs, or using automated reminder systems.
- *Behavioral interventions* focus on changing specific behaviors, typically through use of positive reinforcement (or reward) for increasing desired behaviors, and to a lesser degree punishment for reducing the frequency of undesired behaviors. To be effective behavioral interventions typically require specialized training in behavioral health principles or clinical psychology.
- *Psychosocial interventions* are focused on the comorbidities that often accompany nonadherence (e.g., cognitive-behavioral therapy for depression). Psychoso-

M. E. Hilliard (✉)
Department of Pediatrics, Section of Psychology,
Baylor College of Medicine, Houston, Texas, USA
e-mail: marisa.hilliard@bcm.edu

© Springer International Publishing Switzerland 2015
D. D. Schwartz, M. E. Axelrad, *Healthcare Partnerships for Pediatric Adherence,*
SpringerBriefs in Public Health, DOI 10.1007/978-3-319-13668-4_4

cial interventions do not specifically target adherence, but can be used in concert with explicitly adherence-oriented approaches.

Although there is variability in the format, content, length, and other details of adherence interventions, nearly all meta-analyses and reviews conclude that behavioral and multicomponent interventions tend to have the greatest impact on improving adherence, both for acute (Wu and Roberts 2008) and chronic medical conditions (Dean et al. 2010; Graves et al. 2010; Kahana et al. 2008; Lemanek et al. 2001; Salema et al. 2011) compared to other intervention strategies. That is, interventions were most successful when they included behavioral strategies such as goal-setting, problem-solving, behavioral contracting, contingencies/incentives, and developing behavioral routines, either alone or in combination with other components (e.g., psychological symptoms, health education).

There is some evidence that treating psychosocial factors within a behavioral intervention may boost its effectiveness. A meta-analysis of adherence promotion interventions for youth with type 1 diabetes found that those that have the largest impact on diabetes control tended to be multicomponent interventions that focused on adherence behaviors in combination with emotional, social, or family processes related to diabetes management (Hood et al. 2010). Clinical experience suggests that when patients present with more severe psychological difficulties such as major depression or bipolar disorder, the mental illness almost always needs to be treated first, before nonadherent behaviors can begin to be addressed.

Other beneficial components of interventions include: making interventions disease-specific (Wysocki et al. 2006); tailoring the content to youths' developmental level; including family members in the intervention; and making interventions more accessible by delivering them at home, in school, or via technology (Salema et al. 2011). Interventions focusing on education alone have been found least effective in changing adherence behavior.

Of note, the patterns that emerge for improving adherence largely translate to improvements in health outcomes as well (Graves et al. 2010; Pai and McGrady 2014). For group comparison studies, Graves et al. reported small but significant effects of adherence interventions on glycemic control in type 1 diabetes ($d=0.28$) and BMI in obesity ($d=0.10$), and large effects on pulmonary function in asthma ($d=1.01$) and in overall healthcare utilization ($d=1.41$). Moreover, these health benefits remained significant on subsequent follow-up. Moderate-to-large effects on health were found for single-subject designs ($d=0.74$) that also persisted on follow-up ($d=0.87$)(specific illness variables not reported). Taken together, these findings provide relatively strong support for the health benefits of adherence-focused interventions.

Family-Focused Interventions

Historically, behavioral interventions delivered to youth with chronic conditions and to their families (e.g., a parent or the family unit as a whole) have been among the most successful in improving adherence behaviors. Given the documented importance of collaborative, age-appropriate family involvement in youths' disease management and the risks associated with conflictual or uninvolved family relationships (Naar-King et al. 2013; Reed-Knight et al. 2011; Wysocki et al. 2008), the importance of intervening at the family level is unsurprising. Effective family interventions to improve adherence to a range of chronic condition treatment regimens include *family teamwork interventions* that teach disease-related problem-solving and family communication skills (Anderson et al. 1999; Duncan et al. 2013) and *family systems therapy* interventions that target maladaptive family interactions (Wysocki et al. 2006; Gray et al. 2011). Family-level interventions tend to be most effective when they are tailored to the specific chronic illness and the issues that arise around illness management.

Recent Innovations in Adherence Interventions

Electronic Monitoring Feedback A major focus of recent intervention studies has been the integration of routine adherence monitoring with feedback about adherence patterns to the patient and family (Herzer et al. 2012). In this approach, electronic monitors including pill bottles, inhalers, glucometers, or other tracking devices are used to record patients' medication adherence, and the healthcare provider or interventionist reviews the objective adherence data with the patient. The goal of electronic monitoring feedback is to allow patients and families to examine their own adherence data to identify behavioral patterns, generate solutions, and observe their progress over time (Herzer et al. 2012).

Electronic monitoring feedback is increasingly included as one piece of larger multicomponent behavioral interventions targeting adherence (e.g., problem-solving, cognitive behavioral therapy, behavioral contracts and incentives). Evidence from clinical trials for the use of electronic monitoring feedback across pediatric populations is mounting, with the most support for improved adherence among youth with asthma (Burgess et al. 2010; Chan et al. 2013; Otsuki et al. 2009; Rohan et al. 2013). Improved adherence among youth with epilepsy (Modi et al. 2013) as well as case studies using this approach with patients with Fanconi Anemia (Hilliard et al. 2011), ulcerative colitis, spina bifida, cystic fibrosis, Crohn's disease (Cortina et al. 2013), end stage renal disease, post-kidney transplant, (Herzer et al. 2012), and asthma (Spaulding et al. 2012) further support this as a promising new intervention strategy.

Motivational Interviewing (MI) MI as a strategy for promoting adherence has also been an increasing focus of empirical investigation in recent years (Duff and Latchford 2010; Gayes and Steele 2014; Suarez and Mullins 2008). A communication style more than a manualized intervention, MI provides a way for healthcare providers to discuss potential health behavior changes with patients and families (Suarez and Mullins 2008). Using this approach, interventionists provide an opportunity for patients to consider how engaging in particular health behaviors (e.g., medication adherence) would or would not align with their personal goals. The ultimate aim of this communication style is for the patient to verbalize and act on personal motivation to engage in the health behaviors. As MI approaches are highly patient-centered, it has been suggested that they may be particularly helpful during times when motivations and goals are conflicting and in flux, for example in adolescence or during the transition into adulthood (Powell et al. 2014).

Results of MI interventions to date have been mixed. A recent meta-analysis of MI interventions for pediatric adherence across a range of conditions found a small but significant overall effect size (g = 0.28)(Gayes and Steele 2014). Moreover, while direct improvements in adherence in response to MI are not always evident, other benefits such as increases in motivation and readiness to adhere to medications, improvements in health-related quality of life, and decreases in symptoms have been reported for adolescents with asthma (Riekert et al. 2011; Seid et al. 2012), diabetes (Channon et al. 2007), and HIV (Naar-King et al. 2010). The potential utility of MI to promote treatment adherence among youth with other conditions (e.g., cystic fibrosis, obesity) has been emphasized (Gayes and Steele 2014) and ongoing research in this area will continue to evaluate the impact on adherence to treatment recommendations (Bean et al. 2012; Flattum et al. 2009; MacDonnell et al. 2012).

Like electronic monitoring feedback, MI is often integrated into multicomponent interventions (Flattum et al. 2009; Seid et al. 2012). There is evidence that its incorporation may enhance treatment by improving patient participation and retention in intervention (Powell et al. 2014), an important issue given high rates of treatment attrition (Skelton and Beech 2011). For example, Bean et al. (2014) used a two session MI intervention with adolescents in a multidisciplinary treatment program for pediatric overweight/obesity. Participants remained in treatment longer and had better long-term follow-up. Thus, a primary value of MI approaches might be to help maximize the effectiveness of other evidence-based interventions.

Provider-Based Intervention Delivery

There are many ways in which pediatricians and other healthcare providers can foster adherence in their patients. Providers assess patient and family knowledge and understanding of the disease and its treatment, and provide ongoing education as the disease course changes and children grow and develop. When possible, simplifying the treatment regimen can reduce barriers to adherence such as cost and treatment burden (Wolf et al. 2011).

In order for healthcare provider-based adherence promoting interventions to be effective, providers must be trained in the intervention skills and protocols. Thus, researchers have begun evaluating the outcomes of training providers to conduct basic behavioral interventions traditionally delivered by behavioral health specialists. For example, Rohan and colleagues (2013) conducted a pilot study of provider training in electronic monitoring feedback, in which they trained pediatric pulmonologists to routinely collect and discuss electronic adherence data from their patients with asthma. The pulmonologists participated in a single training session plus individual supervision following patient visits for several months. Short-term improvements in children's adherence to preventive asthma medications were reported, compared to patients whose providers did not use this approach.

Researchers have also evaluated the impact of training pediatric healthcare providers in MI (Bean et al. 2012; Lozano et al. 2010). In both published examples of MI training, 6–9 hours of group MI training were conducted, including didactic teaching about the MI philosophy and specific skills, review and discussion of video vignettes, and in vivo role-play practice with feedback from the trainers. Lozano and colleagues (2010) also observed participants delivering MI, and provided feedback after 3 months of using MI in practice. In both studies, improvements were reported in providers' understanding of MI and in using MI skills in clinical encounters. Across both intervention types, the provider trainings were noted to be feasible and acceptable to clinicians.

Other interventions to teach providers effective communication skills and promote patient-centered care have been developed and investigated in pediatric and adult healthcare settings (Nobile and Drotar 2003; Zolnierek and DiMatteo 2009). These interventions tend to result in improvements in the patient-provider relationship, and in observer ratings of provider communication skills and patient-centeredness (e.g., demonstrating empathy, asking questions, encouraging the patient/family to participate in medical decision-making). To a lesser degree, some benefits have been reported in terms of adherence behaviors or health outcomes; however, such studies with pediatric health care providers have been limited (Birk et al. 2005; Dwamena et al. 2012; Nobile and Drotar 2003).

Studies suggest that there is a pressing need for these types of interventions. Youth with chronic conditions often report that they have difficulty receiving understandable answers to health questions and that they feel under-involved in medical decisions (Byczkowski et al. 2010; Van Staa 2011), factors that can influence their participation in medical self-care. Extending communication skills training to pediatric providers may help address this concern. Communication skills training may also be especially important for working with families from racial/ethnic or socioeconomic minority backgrounds, who frequently report dissatisfaction with provider communication and rapport-building, as we discuss in more detail in Chap. 9.

Taken together, these results suggest a promising future for disseminating both electronic monitoring feedback and MI into clinical research and practice for pediatric adherence intervention via well-trained healthcare providers. However, these relatively brief trainings are often insufficient for providers to reach competence in the approach (e.g., Bean et al. 2012), and there are no data to date on long-term effects or direct effects on patient outcomes. These approaches may therefore be most suitable as "universal-level" interventions (Kazak 2006) focused on improving the healthcare provided to all patients, but they are unlikely to be very effective for many patients and families at higher risk, who are at higher risk and face more barriers with adherence and illness control.

Technology, eHealth, and mHealth

The use of technology in adherence intervention research is an area of rapid growth. Technology-based interventions include delivery of strategies to promote adherence via the internet (eHealth) or electronic mobile devices such as with text messaging or smartphone applications (mHealth). Noted benefits of using technology to deliver adherence promotion interventions include reaching youth through a medium with which they are familiar and already engaged, potential for individualization, and the ability to assess adherence as well as intervene (Wu and Hommel 2014).[1]

Evidence for technology-based interventions is building, with encouraging findings for using the internet or mobile devices to deliver behaviorally-based interventions to promote treatment adherence for youth with various chronic conditions (Cushing and Steele 2010; Herbert et al. 2013; Stinson et al. 2009; Wu and Hommel 2014). Like their in-person counterparts, technology-based adherence interventions that emphasize behavioral components have more consistent beneficial effects on adherence outcomes (Cushing and Steele 2010). In addition, recommendations include integrating the technology with a human interaction, such as using eHealth to supplement in-person intervention, or including a face-to-face meetings with a health coach at the start of a mobile intervention, as the supportiveness and accountability of human contact can help increase participants' motivation and engagement with the technology (Mohr et al. 2011).

In the past five years, technology interventions have been shown to result in improvement in adherence to medical treatments for many pediatric chronic conditions, including type 1 diabetes (Herbert et al. 2013; Mulvaney et al. 2010), asthma (Gustafson et al. 2014; Searing and Bender 2012), HIV (Dowshen et al. 2012; Naar-King et al. 2013; Shegog et al. 2012), cystic fibrosis (Marciel et al. 2010), cancer (Kato et al. 2008), sickle cell disease (Creary et al. 2014), post-liver transplant (Miloh et al. 2009), and systemic lupus erythematosus (Ting et al. 2012). Medication or treatment reminders via text message are among the most common types of technology interventions (Cole-Lewis and Kershaw 2010). Although the use of technology does not necessarily equate to improvements in adherence, it may increase the accessibility and reach of adherence promotion interventions and thus holds the potential to increase the likelihood of adherence behaviors occurring in their natural or recommended times and places.

Targeting Interventions to the Highest Risk Patients

Patients at the highest risk for disparities in adherence and health outcomes tend to be poor and to come from racial and ethnic minority backgrounds (see Chap. 8 and 9). They also account for a very large proportion of all health expenditures, largely

---

[1] Although the electronic monitoring feedback interventions described above by definition use technological tools to monitor adherence, the feedback portion is typically delivered in person and thus is distinct from the interventions discussed in this section.

through expensive hospitalizations for illness crises. Many of these hospitalizations result from nonadherence and therefore may be preventable to some degree (Schwartz et al. 2010). With the changing economic climate impacting healthcare, the need to reduce healthcare costs is ever more evident. To begin to address this issue, adherence promotion interventions have been developed that focus on improving health, and thus reducing healthcare costs, among the patients at highest risk for poor health outcomes. Targeting resources to the patients in greatest need is also necessitated by the relative paucity of available services (Kazak 2006).

In order to deliver care to the patients in greatest need of adherence promotion intervention, patients may be identified in a number of ways, including physical signs of poor illness control, multiple hospitalizations for disease complications, significant psychosocial distress, or behavioral measures of non-adherence. Among youth with epilepsy, Modi et al. (2013) used electronic adherence monitoring to assess patients' average weekly adherence rates, and triaged patients to different levels of adherence intervention accordingly. Similarly, Gamble et al. (2011) identified patients with low adherence via pharmacy refill records prior to being enrolled in an adherence promotion intervention. Many of these interventions emphasize preventive intervention early in the disease course, which is likely to be an important component of adherence promotion.

Once patients are identified as being in need of intervention, evidence-based treatments have been adapted to target adherence behaviors for specific diseases. For example, Behavioral Family Systems Therapy is a well-validated, multicomponent intervention that has been tailored for the unique issues and challenges of managing type 1 diabetes, particularly among youth with glycemic control well outside the recommended range (Wysocki et al. 2008).

Multisystemic Interventions Many of the patients at highest risk have multiple comorbid risk factors that may span individual, family, and socioeconomic levels. A number of recent interventions focus on a more multilevel approach to care, often using a home- and community-based approach. Multisystemic therapy (MST) is an evidence-based treatment approach for youth at high risk that addresses individual and family factors within the broader contexts (e.g., school, healthcare system) in which they exist. MST interventions have resulted in significant improvements in adherence and health outcomes for youth with type 1 diabetes who have chronically poor metabolic control (Ellis et al. 2005) and for poorly adherent youth with HIV (Ellis et al. 2006; Letorneau et al. 2013).

Multisystemic interventions are highly promising and likely necessary to advance the effectiveness of adherence interventions, given the multifactorial nature of many adherence difficulties. However, they tend to be resource-intensive and may not always be feasible to implement on a wide scale. An important area for future clinical research is to demonstrate that these interventions can be cost-effective. In important recent work, Harris and colleagues (2013) have demonstrated the feasibility and economic benefits of intensive individualized intervention implemented in clinical practice for the costliest, highest risk youth with a range of chronic conditions. The *Novel Interventions in Children's Healthcare* (NICH) program provides intensive in-home interventions for youth who are repeatedly hospitalized for preventable health problems, with the goal of improving adherence by address-ing barriers to care in all parts of the child's environment. NICH interventionists provide care coordination, case management, and family-based problem-solving therapy, maintaining close contact with the family and acting as a liaison between the youth, the family, healthcare providers, community agencies and schools. Pre-liminary data show that the program results in substantial reduction of hospitaliza-tions and healthcare costs (Harris et al., 2014).

Summary and Conclusions: Adherence Promotion in Clinical Practice

After several decades of research, we have a good understanding of what works to treat nonadherence, and why. Effective interventions tend to use behavioral strate-gies, incorporate some patient education, address comorbidities, and involve the family in care. They also may focus on improving provider communication with patients, (see Chap. 9).

In a recent editorial introducing a special issue on adherence in the *Journal of Pediatric Psychology*, Stark (2013) offered a number of additional conclusions. First, she suggested that recent studies indicate that treatment benefits do not ap-pear to outlast the duration of intervention, suggesting the need for boosters or other ongoing processes to foster adherence and detect nonadherence in the longer term. Second, she highlighted that patients in real-world settings differ from carefully selected study participants in that they are characterized by co-morbidities and com-plexities that are winnowed out in well-controlled research. Thus, providers should be wary of generalizing study findings to clinical settings; and indeed, empirically-supported treatments are only one part of evidence-based practice, along with pa-tient/family preferences, and clinical expertise (Spring 2008). However, the recent move toward multi-component interventions and intervention studies conducted in the field (e.g., Harris et al. 2013) is likely to build the evidence base for empirically-supported interventions for more children and families.

Table 4.1 summarizes the mean effect sizes for different adherence interven-tions as reported in various recent meta-analyses. Effects range from small to large depending on intervention type, sample characteristics, and study design (single-subject versus group), although overall the effects seem to fall primarily in the small to medium range. As noted above, medium effects can be clinically meaningful, as evidenced by the improvements in health outcomes noted by Graves et al. The large effects found for single-subject designs are also encouraging, as these studies may better reflect the actualities of everyday clinical practice. However, it should be noted that the large reported effects might reflect publication bias (Graves et al. 2010).

Table 4.1 Mean effect sizes reported in adherence intervention meta-analyses

Intervention	M effect size	Categorization	Reference
Overall	0.20–0.29	Small	Pai and McGrady 2014
	0.34	Small	Kahana et al. 2008
	0.58	Medium	Graves et al. 2010
	1.53*	Large	
Behavioral	0.54	Medium	Kahana et al. 2008
	0.11	Small	Wu and Roberts 2008
Multi-component	0.51	Medium	Kahana et al. 2008
	0.60–1.33	Medium-Large	Wu and Roberts 2008
Educational	0.16	Small	Kahana et al. 2008
	−0.42†	Medium	Wu and Roberts 2008

Note: Effect size categorization: 0.20=small; 0.50=medium; 0.80=large (Cohen 1992)
*Single-subject designs. All other effect sizes are for group studies
† Negative effect size indicates outcomes were better in control group than intervention group

References

Anderson B, Brackett J, Ho J, Laffel LM. An office-based intervention to maintain parent-adolescent teamwork in diabetes management. Impact on parent involvement, family conflict, and subsequent glycemic control. Diabetes Care. 1999;22:713–21.

Bean MK, Biskobing D, Francis GL, Wickham E. Motivational interviewing in health care: Results of a brief training in endocrinology. J Grad Med Educ. 2012;4:357–61.

Bean MK, Powell P, Quinoy A, Ingersoll K, Wickham EP III. Motivational interviewing targeting diet and physical activity improves adherence to paediatric obesity treatment: results from the MI Values randomized controlled trial. Pediatr Obes. 2014. Early View (Online Version of Record published before inclusion in an issue). http://dx.doi.org/10.1111/j.2047-6310.2014.226.x.

Birk NA, Cabana MD, Clark NM. Teachable moments: improving pediatric asthma outcomes through physician education. Expert Rev Pharmacoecon Outcomes Res. 2005;5:287–96.

Burgess SW, Sly PD, Devadason SG. Providing feedback on adherence increases use of preventive medication by asthmatic children. J Asthma. 2010;47:198–201.

Byczkowski TL, Kollar LM, Britto MT. Family experiences with outpatient care: do adolescents and parents have the same perceptions? J Adol Health. 2010;47:92–8.

Chan AHY, Reddel HK, Apter A, Eakin M, Riekert K, Foster JM. Adherence monitoring and e-health: how clinicians and researchers can use technology to promote inhaler adherence for asthma. J Allergy Clin Immunol Pract. 2013;1:445–54.

Channon SJ, Huws-Thomas MV, Rollnick S, Hood K, Cannings-John RL, Rogers C, Gregory JW. A multicenter randomized controlled trial of motivational interviewing in teenagers with diabetes. Diabetes Care. 2007;30:1390–5.

Cohen J. A power primer. Psychol Bull. 1992;112:155–9.

Cole-Lewis H, Kershaw T. Text messaging as a tool for behavior change in disease prevention and management. Epidemiol Rev. 2010;32:56–69.

Cortina S, Somers M, Rohan JM, Drotar D. Clinical effectiveness of comprehensive psychological intervention for nonadherence to medical treatment: a case series. J Pediatr Psychol. 2013;38:649–63.

Creary SE, Gladwin MT, Byrne M, Hildesheim M, Krishnamurti L A pilot study of electronic directly observed therapy to improve hydroxyurea adherence in pediatric patients with sickle cell disease. Pediatr Blood Cancer 2014. doi 10.1002/pbc.24931.

Cushing CC, Steele RG. A meta-analytic review of eHealth interventions for pediatric health promoting and maintaining behaviors. J Pediatr Psychol. 2010;35:937–49.

Dean AJ, Walters J, Hall A. A systematic review of interventions to enhance medication adherence in children and adolescents with chronic illness. Arch Dis Child. 2010;95:717–23.

Dowshen N, Kuhns LM, Johnson A, Holoyda BJ, Garofalo R. Improving adherence to antiretroviral therapy for youth living with HIV/AIDS: a pilot study using personalized, interactive, daily text message reminders. J Med Internet Res. 2012;14(2):e51.

Duff AJA, Latchford GJ. Motivational interviewing for adherence problems in cystic fibrosis. Pediatr Pulmonol. 2010;45:211–20.

Duncan CL, Hogan MB, Tien KJ, Graves MM, Chorney JM, Zettler MD, Koven L, Wilson NW, Dinakar C, Portnoy J. Efficacy of a parent-youth teamwork intervention to promote adherence in pediatric asthma. J Pediatr Psychol. 2013;38:617–28.

Dwamena F, Holmes-Rovner M, Gaulden CM, Jorgenson S, Sadigh G, Sikorskii A, Lewin S, Smith RC, Coffey J, Olomu A. Interventions for providers to promote a patient-centered approach in clinical consultations. Cochrane Database Syst Rev. 2012 Issue 12. Art. No.: CD003267. doi: 10.1002/14651858.CD003267.pub2.

Ellis DA, Frey MA, Naar-King S, Templin T, Cunningham P, Cakan N. Use of multisystemic therapy to improve regimen adherence among adolescents with type 1 diabetes in chronic poor metabolic control: a randomized controlled trial. Diabetes Care. 2005;28:1604–10.

Ellis DA, Naar-King S, Cunningham PB, Secord E. Use of multisystemic therapy to improve antiretroviral adherence and health outcomes in HIV-infected pediatric patients: evaluation of a pilot program. AIDS Patient Care STDS. 2006;20:112–21.

Flattum C, Friend S, Neumark-Sztainer D, Story M. Motivational interviewing as a component of a school-based obesity prevention program for adolescent girls. J Am Diet Assoc. 2009;109:91–4.

Gamble J, Stevenson M, Heaney LG. A study of a multi-level intervention to improve non-adherence in difficult to control asthma. Respiratory Med. 2011;105:1308–15.

Gayes LA, Steele RG. A meta-analysis of motivational interviewing interventions for pediatric health behavior change. J Consult Clin Psychol. 2014;82:521–35.

Graves MM, Roberts MC, Rapoff M, Boyer A. The efficacy of adherence interventions for chronically ill children: A meta-analytic review. J Pediatr Psychol. 2010;35:368–82.

Gray WN, Janicke DM, Fennell EB, Driscoll DC, Lawrence RM. Piloting behavioral family systems therapy to improve adherence among adolescents with HIV: a case series intervention study. J Health Psychol. 2011;16:828–42.

Gustafson D, Wise M, Bhattacharya A, Pulvermacher A, Shanovich K, Phillips B, Lehman E, Chinchilli V, Hawkins R, Kim J. The effects of combining web-based eHealth with telephone nurse case management for pediatric asthma control: a randomized controlled trial. J Medical Internet Research. 2014;14:e101.

Harris MA, Spiro K, Heywood M, Wagner DV, Hoehn D, Hatten A, Labby D. Novel interventions in children's health care (NICH): innovative treatment for youth with complex medical conditions. Clin Pract Pediatr Psychol. 2013;1:137–45.

Harris MA, Wagner DV, Heywood M, Hoehn D, Bahia H, Spiro K. Youth repeatedly hospitalized for DKA: proof of concept for novel interventions in children's healthcare (NICH). Diabetes Care. 2014;37(6):e125–6.

Herbert L, Owen V, Pascarella L, Streisand R Text message interventions for children and adolescents with type 1 diabetes: a systematic review. Diabetes Technol Ther. 2013;15(5):362–70.

Herzer M, Ramey C, Rohan J, Cortina S. Incorporating electronic monitoring feedback into clinical care: a novel and promising adherence promotion approach. Clin Child Psychol Psychiatry. 2012;17:505–18.

Hilliard ME, Ramey C, Rohan JM, Drotar D, Cortina S. Electronic monitoring feedback to promote adherence in an adolescent with Fanconi Anemia. Health Psychol. 2011;30:503–9.

Hood KK, Peterson CM, Rohan JM, Drotar D. Interventions with adherence-promoting components in pediatric type 1 diabetes: meta-analysis of their impact on glycemic control. Diabetes Care. 2010;33:1658–64.

Kahana S, Drotar D, Frazier T. Meta-analysis of psychological interventions to promote adherence to treatment in pediatric chronic health conditions. J Pediatr Psychol. 2008;33:590–611.

Kato PM, Cole, Steve W, Bradlyn AS, Pollock BH. A video game improves behavioral outcomes in adolescents and young adults with cancer: a randomized trial. Pediatrics. 2008;122(2):305–17.

Kazak AE. Pediatric Psychosocial Preventative Health Model (PPPHM): research, practice and collaboration in pediatric family systems medicine. Fam Sys Health. 2006;24:381–95.

Lemanek KL, Kamps J, Chung NB. Empirically supported treatments in pediatric psychology: regimen adherence. J Pediatr Psychol. 2001;26:253–75.

Letorneau EJ, Ellis DA, Naar-King S, Chapman JE, Cunningham PB, Fowler S. Multisystemic therapy for poorly adherence youth with HIV: Results from a pilot randomized controlled trial. AIDS Care. 2013;25(4):507–14.

Lozano P, McPhillips HA, Hartzler B, Robertson AS, Runkle C, Scholz KA, Stout JW, Kieckhefer GM. Randomized trial of teaching brief motivational interviewing to pediatric trainees to promote healthy behaviors in families. Arch Pediatr Adolesc Med. 2010;164:561–6.

MacDonnell K, Brogan K, Naar-King S, Ellis D, Marshall S. A pilot study of motivational interviewing targeting weight-related behaviors in overweight or obese African American adolescents. J Adolesc Health. 2012;50:201–3.

Miloh T, Annunziato R, Arnon R, et al. Improved adherence and outcomes for pediatric liver transplant recipients by using text messaging. Pediatrics. 2009;124:e844–e50.

Modi AC, Guilfoyle SM, Rausch J. Preliminary feasibility, acceptability, and efficacy of an innovative adherence intervention for children with newly diagnosed epilepsy. J Pediatr Psychol. 2013;38:605–16.

Mohr DC, Cujipers P, Lehman K. Supportive accountability: a model for providing human support to enhance adherence to eHealth interventions. J Med Internet Res. 2011;13:e30.

Mulvaney SA, Rothman RL, Wallston KA, Lybarger C, Dietrich MC. An internet-based program to improve self-management in adolescents with type 1 diabetes. Diabetes Care. 2010;33:602–4.

Naar-King S, Parsons JT, Murphy D, Kolmodin K, Harris DR. A multisite randomized trial of motivational intervention targeting multiple risks in youth living with HIV: initial effects on motivation, self-efficacy, and depression. J Adolesc Health. 2010;46:422–8.

Naar-King S, Outlaw AY, Sarr M, Parsons JT, Belzer M, MacDonnell K, Tanney M, Ondersma SJ. Motivational enhancement system for adherence (MESA): pilot randomized trial of a brief computer-delivered prevention intervention for youth initiating antiretroviral treatment. J Pediatr Psychol. 2013;38:638–48.

Nobile C, Drotar D. Research on the quality of parent-provider communication in pediatric care: implications and recommendations. J Dev Behav Pediatr. 2003;24:279–90.

Otsuki M, Eakin MN, Rand CS, Butz AM, Hsu VD, Zuckerman IH, Ogborn J, Bilderback A, Riekert KA. Adherence feedback to improve asthma outcomes among inner-city children: a randomized trial. Pediatrics. 2009;124:1513–21.

Pai ALH, McGrady M. Systematic review and meta-analysis of psychological interventions to promote treatment adherence in children, adolescents, and young adults with chronic illness. J Pediatr Psychol. 2014;39:918–31.

Powell PW, Hilliard ME, Anderson BJ. Motivational interviewing to promote adherence behaviors in pediatric type 1 diabetes. Curr Diab Rep. 2014;14:531.

Rapoff MA. Adherence to pediatric medical regimens. 2nd ed. New York: Springer; 2010.

Reed-Knight B, Lewis JD, Blount RL. Association of disease, adolescent, and family factors with medication adherence in pediatric inflammatory bowel disease. J Pediatr Psychol. 2011;36:308–17.

Riekert KA, Borrelli B, Bilderback A, Rand CS. The development of a motivational interviewing intervention to promote medication adherence among inner-city, African-American adolescents with asthma. Patient Educ Couns. 2011;82:117–22.

Rohan JM, Drotar D, Perry AR, McDowell K, Malkin J, Kercsmar C. Training health care providers to conduct adherence promotion in pediatric settings: an example with pediatric asthma. Clin Pract Pediatr Psychol. 2013;1:314–25.

Salema NM, Elliott RA, Glazebrook C. A systematic review of adherence-enhancing interventions in adolescents taking long-term medicines. J Adolesc Health. 2011;49:455–66.

Schwartz DD, Cline VD, Hansen J, Axelrad ME, Anderson BJ. Early risk factors for nonadherence in pediatric type 1 diabetes: a review of the recent literature. Curr Diabetes Rev. 2010;6:167–83.

Searing DA, Bender BG. Short message service (SMS) for asthma management: a pilot study utilizing text messaging to promote asthma self-management. J Allergy Clin Immunol 2012;129:AB142.

Seid M, D'Amico EJ, Varni JW, Munafo JK, Britto MT, Kercsmar CM, Drotar D, King EC, Darbie L. The in vivo adherence intervention for at risk adolescents with asthma: report of a randomized pilot trial. J Pediatr Psychol. 2012;37:390–403.

Shegog R, Markham CM, Leonard AD, Bui TC, Paul ME. "+ Click": pilot of a web-based training program to enhance ART adherence among HIV-positive youth. AIDS Care. 2012;24:310–8.

Skelton JA, Beech BM. Attrition in pediatric weight management: a review of the literature and new directions. Obes Rev. 2011;12:e273–e81.

Spaulding SA, Devine KA, Duncan CL, Wilson NW, Hogan MB. Electronic monitoring and feedback to improve adherence in pediatric asthma. J Pediatr Psychol. 2012;37:64–74.

Spring B. Health decision making: lynchpin of evidence-based practice. Med Decis Making. 2008;28:866–74.

Stark L. Introduction to the Special Issue on Adherence in Pediatric Medical Conditions. J Pediatr Psychol. 2013;38:589–94.

Stinson J, Wilson R, Gill N, Yamada J, Holt J. A systematic review of internet-based self-management interventions for youth with health conditions. J Pediatr Psychol. 2009;34:495–510.

Suarez M, Mullins S. Motivational interviewing and pediatric health behavior interventions. J Dev Behav Pediatr. 2008;29:417–28.

Ting TV, Kudalkar D, Nelson S, Cortina S, Pendl J, Budhani S, Neville J, Taylor J, Huggins J, Drotar D, Brunner HI. Usefulness of cellular text messaging for improving adherence among adolescents and young adults with systemic lupus erythematosus. J Rheumatol. 2012;39:174–9.

Van Staa A. Unraveling triadic communication in hospital consultations with adolescents with chronic conditions: The added value of mixed methods research. Patient Educ Couns. 2011;82:455–64.

Wolf MS, Curtis LM, Waite K, Bailey SC, Hedlund LA, Davis TC, Shrank WH, Parker RM, Wood AJJ. Helping patients simplify and safely use complex prescription regimens. Arch Intern Med. 2011;171:300–5.

Wu YP, Hommel KA. Using technology to assess and promote adherence to medical regimens in pediatric chronic illness. J Pediatr. 2014; doi:10.1016/j.peds.2013.11.013.

Wu YP, Roberts MC. A meta-analysis of interventions to increase adherence to medication regimens for pediatric otitis media and streptococcal pharyngitis. J Pediatr Psychol. 2008;33:789–96.

Wysocki T, Harris MA, Buckloh LM, Mertlich D, Lochrie AS, Taylor A, Sadler M, Mauras N, White NH. Effects of behavioral family systems therapy for diabetes on adolescents' family relationships, treatment adherence, and metabolic control. J Pediatr Psychol. 2006;31:928–38.

Wysocki T, Harris MA, Buckloh LM, Mertlich D, Lochrie AS, Taylor A, Sadler M, White NH. Randomized, controlled trial of behavioral family systems therapy for diabetes: maintenance and generalization of effects on parent-adolescent communication. Behav Ther. 2008;39:33–46.

Zolnierek KBH, DiMatteo MR. Physician communication and patient adherence to treatment: a meta-analysis. Med Care. 2009;47:826–34.

Chapter 5
The Importance of Development: Early and Middle Childhood

Children are not little adults
—Rapoff 2010

Abstract Childhood—roughly the time from birth to age 18 years—is a highly dynamic period characterized as much by change as by continuity. This dynamism can present a significant challenge to pediatric illness management above and beyond the challenges faced by adults with chronic illness. Managing a chronic illness in a child is often a moving target—once one aspect of managing the disease seems to have stabilized, another facet emerges. Adjusting family management to the child's development level is therefore critically important. If healthcare providers are to be able to provide truly effective guidance, it is crucial for them to understand the ways in which families adapt to and manage a child's chronic illness over the course of development. In this chapter we discuss family management of illness in the preadolescent years, when management falls primarily or even exclusively on the parent, reviewing some of the common developmental trends and their implications for chronic illness management.

Family management of pediatric illness is typified by an interaction between a child's (developing) abilities and autonomy and (declining) caregiver support over time. Successful illness management requires maintaining an appropriate balance between child autonomy and parent support calibrated to the child's developmental level. This balance has to be continually re-negotiated as the child matures. However, the progression from parent support to child autonomy is not always linear or smooth, and set-backs can be common. De Civita and Dobkin (2004) give the example of a child with chronic illness who experiences a significant illness exacerbation and becomes more dependent on family support; if increased support is not forthcoming, disease management is likely to suffer.

Other changes in the child's life can also upset this balance. A change in schools, in parents' marital status, the birth of a new sibling, taking on too many other activities or responsibilities, social difficulties, and other new onset of stresses are just some of the events that can create a need for parents to increase their level of management support. More directly, if illness control begins to decline, that is often a sign for the need for greater parent involvement (Wysocki 1997).

© Springer International Publishing Switzerland 2015
D. D. Schwartz, M. E. Axelrad, *Healthcare Partnerships for Pediatric Adherence,*
SpringerBriefs in Public Health, DOI 10.1007/978-3-319-13668-4_5

Age is typically used as a proxy for developmental level. While this is a reasonable rule of thumb, practitioners should be aware that there is significant developmental variability within age groups, so age may not always be the best indicator of maturity (de Civita and Dobkin 2004; Wysocki 1996). More important than age itself are (1) the onset of puberty, which ushers in adolescence, a developmental period qualitatively distinct from earlier childhood, and (2) the transition into young adulthood, particularly when the child leaves home and is more or less on his own. Less critical but still important are the transitions that accompany changes from elementary to middle school, and from middle school to high school.

We begin this chapter with a brief consideration of the role of temperament in setting the stage for children's responses to chronic illness and illness management. The remainder of the chapter then focuses on developmental considerations in illness management in early and middle childhood. Adolescence, which is the time of greatest difficulty in treatment adherence, is the focus of Chap. 6. The transition into early adulthood is a complex issue that is beyond the scope of this volume.

The Role of Temperament

Most parents know that children can come into the world with very different *temperaments*, in-born behavioral and emotional response tendencies that emerge early in life and tend to remain stable throughout the lifespan. Some children are easygoing from day one; they tend to respond positively to new things, adapt easily to their environment, and generally "go with the flow." Other children are difficult and not very adaptable to change; they may present as more irritable and more negative. Still others are emotionally reactive; or shy and inhibited; or extremely active, impulsive, and "on the go." These tendencies often become apparent in toddlerhood and tend to persist to some degree, eventually putting a stamp on an individual's personality. Important dimensions of temperament include reactivity, tendency to approach or withdraw in the face of novelty, and ability to self-regulate (Calkins and Howse 2004), which as we saw in Chap. 2 is so important for successful illness management in later childhood and adolescence.

Temperament is relatively stable, with early child temperament predicting both internalizing and externalizing behavioral disorders later in development (e.g., Hinshaw 2008). Studies have shown that between 20–60 % of variance in temperament is due to genetic influences (Saudino 2005). At the same time, environmental factors—especially parenting—also play a powerful role in shaping these behavioral tendencies. The influence between parenting and temperament is bidirectional, with parenting moderating child temperament, and differences in temperament eliciting different parenting styles (Kiff et al. 2011). Temperament also moderates the effects of environmental stress (Schermerhorn et al. 2013) and parental psychopathology (Jessee et al. 2012) on child behavior. Recent theories go further to suggest that some children may be more susceptible to environmental influences (including parenting) than others (e.g., Belsky and Pluess 2009; Boyce and Ellis 2005), such that more sensitive or reactive children may benefit more from positive parenting but suffer more from ineffective or negative parenting.

It is therefore not surprising that temperament can greatly influence parent-child interactions around adherence. Children who are temperamentally more difficult, fearful, or reactive may resist complying with parent requests to cooperate with illness management. They may respond with avoidance or tears or tantrums, making management "a battleground … [that] will require significant emotional stamina by the parent" (Anderson and Schwartz 2014). In contrast, other children may adapt easily to the changes and challenges posed by adhering to a medical regimen. It is important to recognize that these individual differences in response and reactivity are part of each child's biological inheritance, which can help explain in part why adherence is so difficult for some children but not for others.

Chronic Illness in Early Childhood: Trust and Exploration

Young children lack the abilities and the maturity needed to manage a chronic illness. It goes without saying that illness management in early childhood is the complete responsibility of the parent; the child's role is to comply and cooperate. Gaining this cooperation, however, can prove quite challenging at times.

Infants and Toddlers In the first few years of life, the primary developmental tasks facing the child are to develop trusting bonds with caregivers, explore the environment, and begin to develop a sense of control over one's body. As many caregivers discover, toddlers also begin to develop their own mind and will, and much time is spent exploring behavioral limits and seeing what they can do, influence, and get away with.

One major challenge to adherence at this age is *parent anxiety*. Very young children cannot communicate when they are feeling ill or are otherwise symptomatic, complicating parent management of their illness. Moreover, parents will sometimes change *how* they manage an illness due to anxiety. For example, some parents of children with type 1 diabetes intentionally reduce their child's insulin dose out of fear of hypoglycemia, with detrimental effects on long-term illness control (Patton et al. 2008; Wild et al. 2007). Other parents may struggle to give their children needed injections out of fear of hurting their child, although in the majority of cases this anxiety abates over time (Howe et al. 2011).

Even very young children can recognize when their parent is anxious or fearful, and this tends to increase child resistance (Dahlquist 1999). Thus, child resistance and parent anxiety can reinforce each other in a vicious cycle. Many parents avoid giving their children needed treatments because they fear the battle that will result (Anderson and Schwartz 2014). Parents may also have difficulty getting an active toddler to settle down enough to allow for completion of a management task. Sometimes parents needlessly get into battles they could have avoided. We have worked with many parents who would insist that their toddler come to them to receive a treatment, rather than simply bringing the treatment to the child. The battle over coming when called ends up taking precedence over receiving the treatment itself, which in some cases is completely forgotten.

Feeding issues are especially common in very young children, even in those without a chronic illness (Arts-Rodas 1998). In a child with chronic illness, feeding can become especially fraught. On the one hand, dietary limitations associated with illnesses such as PKU or chronic kidney disease can complicate feeding for children who already have restricted eating patterns. On the other hand, it can be even more stressful for a parent when her child has to eat for medical reasons, for example to ensure caloric intake, or soon after a child with diabetes has received an insulin injection (Anderson and Schwartz 2014). Parent desperation in these instances can lead a child to dig in her heels even more. Feeding problems can often be minimized by (Schwartz et al. 2013):

- Creating a regular schedule for feeding, ideally at times the child is typically hungry
- Avoiding battles around feeding and food
- Making play contingent on first eating

Families who continue to struggle with feeding may need to be referred to a behavioral specialist.

Early School-Age Children: Developing Competence

Parents should continue to have complete responsibility for adherence in early school-age children (roughly ages 3 through 7), although children in this age range will begin to ask more questions and can start to learn some concrete facts about their illness and treatment. As they understand more about the importance of adherence to their health, some children in this age range will begin to take greater interest and become more involved in illness management tasks. Children whose parents encourage questioning and give choices where appropriate (e.g., between two acceptable food choices) may do especially well (Chisholm et al. 2011).

At the same time, children may also begin to ask why *they* have to manage a chronic illness while other children their age do not, and they may complain of unfairness and resist cooperating with management tasks. Children in this age range may also wonder whether the illness is in some way their fault, the result of something they did or a punishment for bad behavior, and this may be especially likely in parents who talk about illness-related variables (like blood sugar values) as "good" or "bad" (Anderson and Schwartz 2014). It is important to help parents become aware that their children may have misconceptions about the cause of their illness, and to help correct any misconceptions they may have.

Entry into preschool or kindergarten carries its own set of challenges and risks. While school management is largely beyond the scope of this volume, it is important to note the importance of notifying and educating school personnel about a child's chronic illness, and working with their child's school to develop an appropriate plan for in-school management (e.g., a 504 Plan; see https://www.nhlbi.nih.gov/files/docs/public/lung/guidfam.pdf).

Older School-Age Children: Where Do I Fit In?

Developmentally, older elementary school children and preteens (roughly, ages 8–11) enter a stage where social comparisons become critical. Children try to figure out how they compare to other children and where they fit in to the group. Social conformity often peaks around age 10 or 11 (Steinberg and Monahan 2007), contributing to child resistance to being different in any way. Children may become ashamed of having a chronic illness, or more immediately of having to manage it, and their peers may begin to tease or bully them for being different. Unfortunately, bullying of children with chronic illness (and other disabilities) can be quite common (Van Cleave and Davis 2006), and is more likely to occur when children are restricted from normal school participation in some way (Sentenac et al. 2011).

Cognitively, many children in this age range are capable of learning the details of their medical regimen, and some are capable of performing management tasks independently. Realizing this, many healthcare providers believe that preparing children to take over illness management should begin around age 10 (Geenen et al. 2003). However, cognitive maturity does not equal emotional maturity or responsibility. Most children in this age range are simply not able to initiate and follow though on management tasks with any reliability, even if they do understand (and can articulate) the importance of doing so. There is solid empirical evidence that when older school-age children are given greater responsibility for illness management, illness control suffers (Wysocki et al. 1996). We will review the evidence and discuss the issue of transfer of responsibility in greater detail in Chap. 10.

Summary

The onus of chronic illness management in early and middle childhood largely falls on the parent, and on other adults—such as school personnel—who have responsibility for the child's welfare during the day. This responsibility can weigh heavily on parents, who experience a lot of stress and anxiety due to fears of hurting their child, inability of the child to communicate about symptoms effectively, and battles over compliance, as well as feelings of guilt for having "caused" their child's illness and worries about the future. Parents—in terms of adherence but also in terms of psychosocial adjustment—should be a primary focus for providers working with these families.

As children get older they develop greater competence in all areas, but they still lack the maturity for taking on responsibility for illness management. Beginning to foster child autonomy by providing some choices at these ages can be beneficial (Chisholm et al. 2011), and participation in self-care tasks in a limited way can be encouraged, but it is important not to push too hard, and to be respectful of children's wishes when they indicate through word or deed that they do not feel ready (Anderson and Schwartz 2014).

References

Anderson BJ, Schwartz DD. Psychosocial and family issues in children with type 1 diabetes. In: Umpierrez G, editor. Therapy for diabetes mellitus and related disorders. 6th ed. Alexandria: American Diabetes Association; 2014. pp. 134–55.

Arts-Rodas D, Benoit D. Feeding problems in infancy and early childhood: identification and management. Paediatr Child Health. 1998;3(1):21–7.

Belsky J, Pluess M. Beyond diathesis stress: differential susceptibility to environmental influences. Psychol Bull. 2009;135:885–908.

Boyce WT, Ellis BJ. Biological sensitivity to context: I. An evolutionary-developmental theory of the origins and functions of stress reactivity. Dev Psychopathol. 2005;17:271–301.

Calkins SM, Howse RB. Individual differences in self-regulation: implications for childhood adjustment. In: Philippot P, Feldman RS, editors. The regulation of emotion. Mahwah: Earlbaum; 2004. p. 307–332.

Chisholm V, Atkinson L, Donaldson C, Noyes K, Payne A, Kelnar C. Maternal communication style, problem-solving and dietary adherence in young children with type 1 diabetes. Clin Child Psychol Psychiatry. 2011;16(3):443–58.

Dahlquist L. Pediatric pain management. 1999. New York: Plenum.

De Civita M Dobkin PL. Pediatric adherence as a multidimensional and dynamic construct, involving a triadic partnership. J Ped Psychol. 2004;29:157–69.

Geenen SJ, Powers LE, Sells W. Understanding the role of health care providers during the transition of adolescents with disabilities and special health care needs. J Adolesc Health. 2003;32(3):225–33.

Hinshaw SP. Developmental psychopathology as a scientific discipline: Relevance to behavioral and emotional disorders of childhood and adolescence. In: Beauchaine TP, Hinshaw SP, editors. Child and adolescent psychopathology. Wiley: Hoboken, NJ: 2008. p. 3–26.

Howe CJ, Ratcliffe SJ, Tuttle A, Dougherty S, Lipman TH. Needle anxiety in children with type 1 diabetes and their mothers. MCN Am J Matern Child Nurs. 2011;36:25–31.

Jessee A, Mangelsdorf SC, Shigeto A, Wong MS. Temperament as a moderator of the effects of parental depressive symptoms on child behavior problems. Soc Dev. 2012;21(3):610–27.

Kiff CJ, Lengua LJ, Zalewski M. Nature and nurturing: parenting in the context of child temperament. Clin Child Fam Psychol Rev. 2011 September; 14(3):251–301.

Patton SR, Dolan LM, Henry R, Powers SW. Fear of hypoglycemia in parents of young children with type 1 diabetes mellitus. J Clin Psychol Med Settings. 2008;15:252–9.

Rapoff MA. Adherence to pediatric medical regimens. 2nd ed. New York: Springer; 2010.

Saudino KJ. Behavioral genetics and child temperament. J Dev Behav Pediatr. 2005; 26(3):214–223.

Schermerhorn AC, Bates JE, Goodnight JA, Lansford JE, Dodge KA, Pettit GS. Temperament moderates associations between exposure to stress and children's externalizing problems. Child Dev. 2013;84(5):1579–93.

Schwartz D, Axelrad M, Anderson B. Psychosocial risk screening of children newly diagnosed with type 1 diabetes: a training toolkit for healthcare professionals. MedEdPORTAL. 2013. www.mededportal.org/publication/9643. Accessed 3 Dec 2015.

Sentenac M, Gavin A, Arnaud C, et al. Victims of bullying among students with a disability or chronic illness and their peers: a cross-national study between Ireland and France. J Adolesc Health. 2011;48:461–6.

Steinberg L, Monahan KC. Age differences in resistance to peer influence. Dev Psychol. 2007;43(6):1531–43.

Van Cleave J Davis MM. Bullying and peer victimization among children with special health care needs. Pediatrics. 2006;118:e1212–9.

Wild D, von Maltzahn R, Brohan E, Christensen T, Clauson P, Gonder-Frederick L. A critical review of the literature on fear of hypoglycemia in diabetes: implications for diabetes management and patient education. Patient Educ Couns. 2007;68:10–15.

Wysocki T. The ten keys to helping your child grow up with diabetes. Alexandria: American Diabetes Association; 1997.

Wysocki T, Taylor A, Hough BS, Linscheid TR, Yeates KO, Naglieri JA. Deviation from developmentally appropriate self-care autonomy: association with diabetes outcomes. Diabetes Care. 1996;19(2):119–25.

Chapter 6
Adherence in Adolescence

Tomorrow's life is too late: live today.
—Martial, Epigrams, bk. I, epig. 15. (A.D. 85)

Abstract An understanding of adolescence and adolescent development is critical for clinicians who wish to be able to help their patients with adherence and illness control. Many teens seem perfectly capable of managing a chronic illness, yet to the surprise of many clinicians, adherence is often at its worst in adolescence, as is chronic illness control. In this chapter we explore the reasons why adherence in adolescence is so challenging and frustrating for patients, parents, and providers alike. We argue that some degree of nonadherence is actually likely to be normative due to the developmental, neurodevelopmental, and cognitive changes of this period, which are almost antithetical to maintaining consistent adherence behaviors. Continued parent involvement will therefore turn out to be a key component of successful illness management in the teenage years. Of course, this involvement is not without its own challenges and costs. We conclude that encouraging a focus on supporting patient autonomy (i.e., volitional behavior) without pushing youth independence (i.e., acting alone) can foster youth development without necessitating a withdrawal of needed parental assistance with illness management.

Adolescents struggle more with adherence than any other age group—in fact, adherence is often at its worst in adolescence. Youth with chronic illness experience declining illness control, higher incidence of serious consequences of nonadherence such as organ graft failure and diabetic ketoacidosis, increased stress and depression, and decreased quality of life. At the same time, they find themselves more on their own with illness management, with less support and involvement from parents, and in many cases parent-child conflict increases. Moreover, illness-management goals may conflict with or impede attainment of the normal goals of adolescent development such as achieving a sense of individuality (Seiffge-Krenke 1998). For these reasons, many health professionals find "that managing the complexity and range of health concerns in adolescents is more challenging than for other age groups" (Sawyer et al. 2007).

© Springer International Publishing Switzerland 2015
D. D. Schwartz, M. E. Axelrad, *Healthcare Partnerships for Pediatric Adherence,*
SpringerBriefs in Public Health, DOI 10.1007/978-3-319-13668-4_6

Adolescence is also a time of significantly increased behavioral risk. In fact, morbidity and mortality in teenagers are primarily attributable to risk-taking and health-risk behaviors such as alcohol and drug use and reckless driving (Kann et al. 2013). In this chapter we argue that these phenomena are related—that nonadherence and risk-taking are *both* largely attributable to the normal neurodevelopmental changes that occur in adolescence, and to the consequent changes that occur in the parent-child relationship. We review the evidence from developmental neurobiology and current theories of risk-taking to develop the case that nonadherence in adolescence can in many circumstances be considered either a direct risk-taking behavior itself, or as the result of developmental factors that contribute to risk-taking.

Adolescence—Definition

Adolescence is a time of dramatic changes—physically, mentally, socially. It is a time of opportunities and new experiences, as teens begin to separate from their parents and spend more time with friends, explore romantic and sexual relationships for the first time, and take more responsibility for themselves and for their lives. Many of the challenges of adolescence provide formative experiences that help prepare the youth for the transition into adulthood.

Adolescence is popularly associated with the teenage years, although most researchers now see the period as lasting longer. The American Academy of Pediatrics defines adolescence as the period from 11 to 21 years of age (https://brightfutures. aap.org/pdfs/Guidelines_PDF/18-Adolescence.pdf). Others have defined the period functionally, as "the period of life that starts with the biological changes of puberty and ends at the time at which the individual attains a stable, independent role in society" (Blakemore and Robbins 2012). Colver and Longwell (2013) suggest that adolescence "should be considered to extend from 11 to 25 years of age" so as to reflect the substantial brain development that occurs during this period. Interestingly, the latter formulation overlaps with what has recently been termed "emerging adulthood." As noted by Arnett (2004), who coined the term, "For today's young people, the road to adulthood is a long one. They leave home at age 18 or 19, but most do not marry, become parents, and find a long-term job until at least their late twenties." Adherence remains quite challenging throughout this period, which encompasses the transition from pediatric to adult care, which is deserving of a volume in its own right; but in this chapter we focus primarily on the period in which most youth are still in their parents' homes, i.e. from puberty until around age 18 or so.

Adherence in Adolescence

Health management habits that are established in adolescence set the stage for later self-management. Nonadherence tends to start in adolescence (Kovacs et al. 1992) and, once established, can persist into adulthood. As noted by Rapoff (2010) in his seminal book on pediatric adherence, adolescents are more likely than younger children or adults to have poorer adherence to their medical regimen regardless of which chronic illness you consider. Worse adherence in adolescence has been documented for youth with asthma, cancer, cystic fibrosis, diabetes, HIV/AIDS, juvenile rheumatoid arthritis, and organ transplant (Rapoff 2010), and other conditions as well.

One challenge to adherence at this stage of development is that physical changes associated with puberty can make illness control more difficult. Growth spurts and hormonal changes can reduce the effectiveness of medication. Changes in the immune system can place organ transplant patients at greater risk for graft failure. For youth with diabetes, hormonal changes can also cause blood sugars to increase while insulin sensitivity decreases (Amiel et al. 1986; Helgeson et al. 2009).

These physical changes can make good illness control an unattainable goal for many teens, even when they complete all management tasks as prescribed. This is especially true when healthcare providers and clinical guidelines establish tight parameters for "good" control. For example, current guidelines for glycemic control in youth with type 1 diabetes recommend maintaining hemoglobin A1c below 7.5% (or below 7% if this can be achieved "without excessive hypoglycemia"; American Diabetes Association 2014), as lower A1c has been associated with reduced risk for complications. The problem is that this is not an achievable goal for many youth with T1D due to factors outside of their control, setting them up for failure and frustration.

These frustrations are compounded when parents and healthcare providers believe that youth are doing less to manage their illness than they actually are. Frustration can lead to burnout, leading many youth to feel "hopeless and helpless" and question whether management is worth all the effort. Some simply give up. Even more concerning, mental illnesses such as depression and anxiety often have their onset in adolescence (Kessler et al. 2005), adding an additional layer of risk for teens with chronic conditions (see Chap. 3).

Normal neurodevelopmental changes that occur post-puberty also contribute to the decline in adherence. Adolescence is associated with an increase in sensation-seeking and reward-seeking behaviors that underlie much general risk-taking in teens. This increase occurs prior to the maturation of cognitive control networks that underlie adult self-regulation, and that help temper impulses toward more immediate gratification. At the same time, there is an increasing shift toward greater independence with less parent oversight, which reaches its peak by later adolescence when many teens can drive, further limiting parents' ability to monitor their behavior. Together, these factors create a "perfect storm" of increased risk-taking and increased opportunities for taking risk, with serious implications for adherence.

Nonadherence as Risk-taking Behavior

Heightened risk taking during adolescence is likely to be normative, biologically driven, and, to some extent, inevitable.—Steinberg 2008.

Risk-taking behavior characterizes adolescence. Of course, not all adolescents are risk takers, but the evidence is clear that risk-taking behavior spikes in adolescence, and the ramifications are profound. According to the Youth Risk Behavior Surveillance study (Kann et al. 2013), the leading causes of morbidity and mortality among youth in the United States are related to six health-risk behaviors: (1) behaviors that contribute to unintentional injuries and violence; (2) tobacco use; (3) alcohol and other drug use; (4) risky sexual behaviors; (5) unhealthy diet; and (6) physical inactivity. As the authors note, "these behaviors frequently are interrelated and are established during childhood and adolescence and extend into adulthood."

In youth with chronic illness, nonadherence to the medical regimen can potentially be added to this list of health-risk behaviors. In fact, in many instances nonadherence can be seen as a risk-*taking* behavior, as has been acknowledged by a number of authors (Bender 2006; Kondryn et al. 2011; Sawyer et al. 2007; Taddeo et al. 2008). Every time someone skips an insulin dose or an immunosuppressive pill entails some risk. This is not to imply that nonadherence is always or even most often intentional, the result of a reasoned decision-making process (e.g., *I'm going to stop taking my Metformin because it isn't helping me anyway*). As noted earlier, nonadherence can often result from a spur of the moment decision not to engage in a specific behavior at a specific time (e.g., *If I miss this one dose, it won't hurt me*). Based on clinical experience, we would argue that these spur-of-the-moment risky decisions are very common among teens who struggle with adherence, and that "nonintentional but volitional" risk behavior (Gerrard et al. 2008) may well be characteristic of teens.

Two Paths to Risk-taking

> When asked, most adolescents say they have no intention of engaging in behaviors that put their health at risk; and yet, when given the opportunity, many of them do.—Gibbons 2008

For teens, risk-taking is often unplanned and opportunistic, a reaction to social circumstances. Many teens will deny having any intention to engage in a risky behavior (such as getting into a car with a drunk driver) yet will acknowledge that they may be *willing* to do so if the situation arises (Gibbons et al. 2005). The propensity to take an opportunity for risk when it arises has been termed *behavioral willingness* (Gibbons et al. 2006). Gibbons, Gerrard, and their colleagues have shown that behavioral willingness is a better predictor of teen health-risk behaviors than behavioral *intentions*, which are typically arrived at through a deliberative, goal-oriented process (Gibbons et al. 1998; Gibbons et al. 2004). On the other hand, behavioral intentions are very strong predictors of health maintenance behaviors, at least in adults (Gibbons 2008).

Behavioral willingness—and risky decision-making in general—appears to be enhanced in social contexts and emotionally exciting situations (Gerrard et al. 2003), i.e., "in the heat of the moment." This brings us back to the "hot" and "cool" systems involved in self-regulation discussed earlier (Metcalf and Mischel 1999). In general, adolescents tend to perform like adults on tasks assessing "cool" decision-making in the laboratory, although risk-taking can even be elicited in the lab when social factors come into play.

In an oft-cited study (Gardner and Steinberg 2005), teens, younger adults, and older adults were asked to play a computer driving game of "chicken." The player accumulated more points the farther the car went, but had to stop at a red light or crash (crashing wiped out all of the points). When a yellow light appeared, "players had to decide how much further to allow the car to move, balancing their desire to accumulate points against the possibility of crashing." The longer the car moved provided the measure of risk-taking. All three groups performed similarly when playing the game alone, but when subjects played the game with other people in the room (the social condition), dramatic differences emerged. The teens played much more riskily than young adults, who performed much more riskily than older adults; moreover, the older adults did not change their play in the social condition at all.

Not all decisions are made on the spur-of-the-moment, of course. In fact, most of the research on health behavior in adults has operated under the assumption that decision-making reflects a reasoned process of weighing possible outcomes and then deciding to act (the behavioral intention) based on expectations of success and the subjective values assigned to each outcome (Cohen 1996).

Based on these findings, Gibbons et al. (1998) postulated that there are two pathways to risk-taking behavior: a "reasoned" pathway in which people acknowledge and accept the possibility of negative outcomes but engage in the behavior anyway, and a "reactive" pathway in which risk-taking results from unexpected opportunities that occur most commonly in social situations. The reasoned pathway (assessed by measuring behavioral intentions) is a stronger predictor of health behaviors, whereas the reactive pathway (assessed by measuring behavioral willingness) is a better predictor of risk behaviors (Gibbons 2008). Reyna and Farley (2006) offer a similar typology of risk-takers, differentiating between *risky deliberators* who rationally weigh the costs and benefits of decisions, and *risky reactors*, who more impulsively take risks. As we will see in the next section, current research in both developmental neurobiology and cognitive psychology support this dual-pathway view.

Clinical Implications of the Dual-pathway Model of Risk It is very important for clinicians to recognize the distinction between "cool" competence and "hot" reactivity in their patients. Healthcare providers will assess their patients' knowledge, understanding, and intentions in the exam room, a cool-system setting where youth are likely to appear more competent and capable then they will be in "real life." A patient may be able to answer all questions about her illness and its management but that does not mean she will be able to complete all management behaviors in the face of competing demands (especially social demands).

On occasion, we have heard clinicians suggest that patients are lying when their intensions don't match up with their behaviors, but theory and research would suggest a different explanation. Most teens are probably being quite honest when they say that they *intend* to take all their medicine, or do a better job following dietary restrictions, etc., but their stated intentions may not capture their *willingness* to deviate from prescribed care if certain opportunities arise. They may also underestimate their willingness to deviate when queried in cool settings. When the hot system is quiescent, the cool system is better able to show what it can do, which can lead adults to overestimate a youth's reasoning potential in other settings. In fact, there is some evidence that children may set overly high goals for themselves in the presence of adults; this has been found for children with asthma and diabetes (Hilliard et al. 1985) and children with cancer (Elkin et al. 1998).

Neurodevelopmental Changes in the Adolescent Brain

Recent evidence from neurodevelopmental and neurobiological research suggests that adolescent risk-taking might be the expectable result of normal maturational processes. Specifically, it has been posited that the greater vulnerability to risk-taking in adolescence results from a "temporal disjunction" between the maturation of two brain systems: a social-emotional network that underlies reward-seeking behavior, which peaks in mid-adolescence, and a cognitive-control network that develops more slowly and only reaches maturity in early adulthood (Steinberg 2010). Evidence for these brain changes is reviewed below, after which the discussion will turn to the implications of these findings for adherence.

It is now understood that the brain goes through substantial changes in adolescence almost as dramatic as in the first few years of life (Colver and Longwell 2013). It is only a slight exaggeration to say that the adolescent is not the same person as he or she was as a child. First, there are changes in the relative distribution of cerebral gray and white matter (Paus et al. 1999; Lenroot and Giedd 2006). Gray matter peaks at the start of adolescence and then declines thereafter, while white matter throughout the brain increases steadily into adulthood, either as the result of increasing myelination, increasing axonal diameter, or both. It is currently unclear whether gray matter is "pruned" or whether increasing myelination converts gray to white, but the important outcome of this process is that brain connectivity increases and neural networks become more efficient and probably take on new functional roles (Giedd 2008; Power et al. 2010). Developmental changes in three processing networks that likely play a role in adherence are discussed below.

The social-emotional reward system In early adolescence there is a dramatic increase in the brain's sensitivity to reward and to social-emotional stimuli. There is a surge in activity of the neurotransmitter dopamine in pathways linking subcortical areas involved in emotion processing (limbic system, especially amygdala) and reward sensitivity (ventral striatum, nucleus accumbens) to the frontal lobes, starting around puberty and increasing through mid- and late-adolescence and then declining thereafter (Galván et al. 2006; Steinberg 2010). Dopamine plays an important role in reward-seeking and motivated behavior, and both human and animal studies show that reward-seeking behaviors increase dramatically after puberty (Steinberg 2010). Moreover, the neural reward system sketched above is especially sensitive to *immediate* reward (McClure et al. 2004), and there is good evidence that a preference for immediate versus delayed reward characterizes many teens (Blakemore and Robbins 2012).

Thus, adolescents appear neurodevelopmentally primed to seek out experiences and engage in behaviors that are immediately rewarding (regardless of whether they may have long-term consequences), and their willingness to do so is highly sensitive to social context (Gerrard et al. 2003). It might even be said that heightened activity in the social-emotional network increases behavioral willingness to take risks (Pomery et al. 2009). It makes evolutionary sense that brain systems that underlie social approach and reward-seeking behavior would spike with the onset of reproductive maturity (Casey et al. 2008).

The cognitive-control system The white matter development that occurs throughout adolescence is especially dramatic in the frontal lobes, which are the last region of the brain to fully mature. The frontal lobes are associated with development of *executive functions* (e.g., planning, organization, working memory) so necessary for self-regulation of behavior. There is clear evidence that executive functions play a critical role in chronic illness management (e.g., Duke and Harris 2014), and more generally in cognitive control. Converging evidence from studies on adolescent brain development strongly supports the conclusion that this period is characterized by a progressive increase in cognitive control (Yurgelun-Todd 2007).

Frontal lobe development is only part of this story. There are also dramatic changes in the *wiring* between frontal control areas and many other regions of the brain, including the limbic system, which is integrally involved in emotion, and the subcortical reward system. The result of this increased functional connectivity is a gradual increase in cognitive control over emotional reactivity, increased ability to delay gratification, and (probably) decreased risk-taking behavior (Olson et al. 2008; Steinberg 2010; but see Berns et al. 2009). As Reyna and Rivers (2008) note, one of the most important developments in adolescence "is the coordination (through improved connectivity) between cortical and subcortical limbic regions—the dance between affect and thinking." However, affect leads this dance into late adolescence, and it is only by the middle of the third decade of life that thinking—cognitive control—takes the lead. This is why car insurance rates are so much higher prior to the age of 25, and why car rental companies often do not let youth younger than 25 rent a car.

Critically, neither social-emotional reactivity or immature frontal lobe functioning by themselves is sufficient to account for increase risk-taking in adolescence; it is the *combination* of these factors, and the temporal gap between their development, that create such a potent vulnerability to risk (Casey et al. 2010; Steinberg 2010). If adolescent risk-taking were simply a result of immature frontal lobe functioning, children would engage in far more risky behavior than adolescents, and this is simply not the case, as evidenced by the alarming spike in risk-taking with the onset of puberty.

An alternative (though not mutually-exclusive) view is that increased activity in the social-emotional network in adolescence may actually *drive* subsequent development of frontal control networks (Bernheim et al. 2013)—in other words, that development of cognitive control may be dependent on experiences gained at least in part through normative risk-taking. In this view, risk behaviors may "present adaptive benefits" by allowing adolescents to gain "skills for survival in absence of parental protection." Of course, the fact that risk-taking may have been evolution-arily adaptive does not necessarily mean that it remains so in the modern world, as the types of risk opportunities have changed (e.g., availability of drugs, guns, and cars) and social constraints have loosened.

Neuroimaging studies of reward processing and decision-making support the developmental lag hypothesis, as they have revealed clear differences in the ways adolescent and adult brains process risk. Adolescents shows different neural activa-tion patterns from adults on executive decision-making tasks (Luna et al. 2010), especially when making decisions about risk (Ernst et al. 2005; Galván et al. 2006). Difference in orbitofrontal cortex activation have especially been noted. Compared to children and adults, adolescents show increased activity in nucleus accumbens relative to orbitofrontal cortex in response to reward (Galván et al. 2006), consistent with the hypothesis that adolescence is characterized by increased reward respon-sivity with relatively diffuse cognitive control. Consistent with the neurobiologi-cal evidence, data from cognitive studies suggests that when risks and rewards are directly compared, rewards win out for teens (but not adults)(Reyna and Farley, 2006). Both cross-sectional and longitudinal neuroimaging studies have demon-strated that adolescents' neural activation patterns become increasingly adult-like as they are able to exhibit more cognitive control (Galván and Rahdar 2013).

The Default Network A third brain system that appears to "come online" during adolescence is the so-called default mode network or default network, a distrib-uted system that includes the frontal lobes, posterior cingulate cortex, and lateral parietal/occipital cortices (especially cuneus and precuneus)(Buckner et al. 2005). Neuroimaging studies have shown that the default network is only sparsely con-nected or fragmented in children (Fair et al. 2008) and likely goes through signifi-cant developmental change throughout adolescence (Blakemore 2012).

The default network becomes activated during resting but awake states and de-activated during goal-directed activity (Broyd et al. 2009). Although its role in cog-nition is currently debated, it is believed to be involved in introspective thought of some sort, possibly including mental imagery, creation and review of mental mod-els and alternative possibilities (Buckner et al. and/or in social cognition (Supekar et al. 2010). There is accruing evidence that the default network might be disrupted by poorly controlled type 1 diabetes (Kaufmann et al. 2011; Perantie et al. 2007), and it has been speculated that default network dysfunction might contribute to adherence difficulties by making it more difficult for individuals to think through possible consequences of their actions (e.g., what might happen if a diabetic teen does not take his insulin; Schwartz et al. 2014).

Clinical Implications of the Neurodevelopmental Evidence

The neurodevelopmental data strongly support the hypothesis that adolescents are driven by increased social-emotional reward sensitivity while lacking the control mechanisms to temper reward-seeking impulses (Galván et al. 2006). Moreover, they are likely to show a preference for immediate over delayed reward (Blakemore and Robbins 2012), and these qualities are heightened in the heat of the moment, when social-emotional rewards are high.

These factors would seem to make it more likely that they would skip a medication dose when asked to go out with friends, or forgo dietary restrictions when snacks are available and parents are not around, than to put those immediately rewarding behaviors aside in favor of the long-term health gains that come from good adherence. To borrow from McClure et al. (2004), the neurodevelopmental data suggest that adolescents are more likely to act like the impatient and self-indulgent grasshopper from Aesop's fable, and less like the patient ant who carefully prepares for the long winter.

Adolescents' increased vulnerability to risk—and the alarming statistics regarding risk-related morbidity and mortality in youth—has led many researchers and professionals with an interest in public health to examine ways in which to reduce these risks and their negative outcomes. This research is discussed more fully in the next section, but for now we will note that one of the few effective approaches to reducing risk has involved reducing *opportunities* to engage in risk through parental monitoring and supervision (Reyna and Farley 2006; cf. Gibbons et al. 2003). Steinberg (2008) sums this view up nicely:

> Strategies such as raising the price of cigarettes, more vigilantly enforcing laws governing the sale of alcohol, expanding adolescents' access to mental-health and contraceptive services, and raising the driving age would likely be more effective in limiting adolescent smoking, substance abuse, pregnancy, and automobile fatalities than strategies aimed at making adolescents wiser, less impulsive, or less shortsighted. Some things just take time to develop, and, like it or not, mature judgment is probably one of them.

Applying this logic to adherence would mean maintaining a relatively high level of vigilance over illness-management behaviors and reducing opportunities for nonadherence. However, it is also important to acknowledge here the opposing view that risk-taking is important for development, that risk behaviors allow adolescents to gain "skills for survival in absence of parental protection" (Bernheim et al. 2013). In this view, reducing risk might reduce opportunities for learning. For example, experiencing an episode of DKA might teach a diabetic teen of the dangers of poor adherence to insulin, with hospitalization providing a "wake-up call" that results in better adherence in the future. Arguing against this idea is the evidence showing that nonadherence in adolescence predicts nonadherence in adulthood. Of course, no one would argue that a teen should be allowed to go into DKA, given the health risks involved, but we have certainly heard the perspective that teens need to be given the freedom to "figure things out for themselves," which, when it comes to illness management, will inevitably involve some risk.

Of course, the fact that risk-taking may have been evolutionarily adaptive does not mean that it remains so in the modern world, as the types of risk opportunities have changed (e.g., drugs, guns, cars) and social constraints have loosened. In the end, it is probably a matter of degree—all parents are faced with the challenge of allowing their children to make mistakes that they can learn from, while still ensuring their health and safety (Sawyer and Aroni 2005). The question becomes how much risk and how many mistakes are allowed before parents step up their level of super-vision. We have here arrived back at one of the central concerns of this book, the tension between parental behavioral control and autonomy support. As we discuss later in this chapter, this tension characterizes changes in the parenting role during adolescence.

Cognitive Factors in Adolescent Decision-making

> Brain systems implicated in basic cognitive processes reach adult levels of maturity by mid-adolescence, whereas those that are active in self-regulation do not fully mature until late adolescence or even early adulthood. In other words, adolescents mature intellectually before they mature socially or emotionally, a fact that helps explain why teenagers who are so smart in some respects sometimes do surprisingly dumb things. –Steinberg 2013

In accordance with a significant reorganization of brain structure and function, changes also occur in the ways adolescents think. Cognitive changes in adolescence are at least as dramatic as neurodevelopmental ones.

Many healthcare providers believe that adolescents who do not follow their regi-men must not understand how to do it correctly, or why it's important to do so. Yet by mid-to-late adolescence, many youth perform similarly to adults on most reason-ing tasks (Steinberg 2010). Unfortunately, we know of no studies directly compar-ing parent and youth knowledge of illness and illness-management (cf. DeWalt and Hinks 2009), although there is no reason to expect that older youths would be less capable of reasoning about illness management than their parents. In fact, research does suggest that teens are most likely to show adult-like patterns of thinking in areas that are most familiar to them (Carey 1988), which is a good characterization of illness management for teens who have been living with the illness for a while.

The problem is that teens do not implement their knowledge consistently. As we saw in previous sections, social-emotional reactivity and immature executive skills help account for of lot of the poor decisions adolescents are famous for. It is like the familiar trope from television. A father asks his teenage son "What were you think-ing?" after the son is caught speeding or drinking or engaged in some other risky behavior, and receives the response: "I wasn't" (http://tvtropes.org/pmwiki/pmwiki.php/Main/WhatWereYouThinking).

However, this is not the whole story. Cognitive factors—i.e., thinking—do also contribute to adolescents' decision-making. Reyna and Farley (2006) review exten-sive evidence that some of adolescents' poor decisions result from using a different *type* of reasoning compared to adults. Specifically, adolescents tend to focus on de-tails when making decisions about engaging in risky behaviors; they weigh the pros and cons, and make (often accurate) judgments about the likelihood of a negative outcome occurring (Reyna et al. 2005). For example, faced with the decision about whether or not to engage in unprotected sex with her boyfriend, an adolescent may correctly reason that the risk of pregnancy or an SDT is relatively low, and hence outweighed by the odds of a pleasurable immediate outcome (Reyna and Farley 2006). Another teen may reason that using a drug "in small doses, just every once in a while … will cause little or no damage to his brain" (NIH Publication No. 13-7589, 2010, revised 2011, 2013). While this supposition may indeed turn out to be true, making it a "good bet" in terms of coldly calculated odds, it is not a bet most adults would make.

Adults are much less likely to engage in this sort of rational deliberation. Instead, adults tend to jump right to the crux of the matter (Reyna 2004), reasoning that the risk of pregnancy or disease or brain damage, however low, is simply not worth it. Reyna and her colleagues argue that adolescents reason based on specific, *verbatim* details (such as the 1 in 20 odds of getting pregnant) and miss the bigger picture, the *gist*, which is what adults tend to base their judgments on. Supportive evidence comes from a clever fMRI study in which participants were asked to press buttons indicating whether an action (such as drinking Drano or setting your hair on fire) was a good idea or a bad idea. Relative to adults, adolescents were slower to make decisions about "bad ideas," and more likely to show activation in dorsolateral prefrontal cortex, a decision-making area of the brain (Baird et al. 2005). The authors suggested that the adults' more automatic responses were driven by "mental images of possible outcomes" (Blakemore and Choudhury 2006), whereas the adolescents were actually *considering* whether drinking Drano etc. was a good idea or not.

Do adolescents engage in this sort of rational risk deliberation when considering whether to omit an insulin dose or forgo a breathing treatment? We don't know (Adams et al. 2004), though given the generality of this tendency to weigh risks, there is no good reason to believe that they wouldn't "consider the odds" when deciding about adherence behaviors as well. Moreover, as it appears that (adult) patients have a general tendency to weigh costs and benefits of adherence (Donovan 1995; Horne and Weinman 1999) or the burden of disease against the burden of treatment (Adams et al. 2004), it seems reasonable to suppose that adolescents would also do so but potentially in a much riskier way, for example by accepting low-odds risks for serious complications of nonadherence (like organ failure or DKA) that adults would rarely consider.

Risk Perceptions

> Contrary to popular wisdom, adolescents see themselves as more vulnerable than adults do, and they typically overestimate important risks.—Reyna and Farley 2006

Perceived vulnerability is an important construct in many models of health behavior (e.g., the Health Belief Model; Janz and Becker 1984). The basic idea is that people will be more likely to engage in an adherence behavior if they believe that there could be a negative outcome to not completing the behavior, and that they are vulnerable to experiencing that outcome. Individuals who do not perceive themselves as vulnerable to a negative outcome are presumed to be more likely to be nonadherent. The research literature is actually equivocal on this point. In a recent meta-analysis, DiMatteo et al. (2007) found that perceived vulnerability (as indexed by disease severity threat) was associated with better adherence only when conditions were less serious (e.g., pharyngitis, asthma). For more serious conditions such as diabetes and end-stage renal disease, parent-perceived severity was associated with worse adherence. Moreover, there was a 14% higher risk for nonadherence in children and youth with objectively poorer health. (Pediatric self-report was not reported.) DiMatteo et al. suggest that adherence may become increasingly difficult when disease status declines, due to feelings of ineffectiveness and (it might be presumed) illness burnout. However, it should be noted that the findings were correlational, making definitive conclusions about causality elusive. Some studies have suggested a curvilinear relationship, with poorer adherence among patients who are asymptomatic and who have more severe symptoms, with adherence being best among patients with active but relatively moderate symptoms (Bender and Klinnert 1998).

When youth risk behavior is discussed in the adherence literature, the focus is often on the notion of adolescent "invulnerability," the idea that "adolescents often believe themselves to be invincible to the consequences of risk-taking behaviors" and therefore are more "susceptible to adherence difficulties" (Kondryn et al. 2011; Taddeo et al. 2008). This view of adolescent invulnerability often leads practitioners to highlight potential consequences and at times even to stress the severest complications in the hopes of "waking the teen up" to the risks he really is facing. The problem is that there is little evidence in support of the invulnerability hypothesis of adolescent risk-taking (Reyna and Farley 2006), and highlighting consequences has been shown to often have the *opposite* of the intended effect, as discussed further below.

Moreover, the evidence suggests that adolescents tend to *overestimate* their vulnerability to risk for many negative outcomes, such as HIV infection or getting lung cancer from smoking (Millstein and Halpern-Felsher 2002). At the same time, however, they tend to underestimate the seriousness of the long-term consequences. As noted by Reyna and Farley (2006), "they think the risk is high, but the consequences are not that bad."

Teenagers do often have what has been termed an *optimistic bias*, a tendency to believe that bad things are much more likely to happen to other people (Gerrard et al. 2008), and the optimistic bias is predictive of poorer adherence (e.g., Patino et al. 2005). However — and this is the crucial point—the optimistic bias is not specific to adolescents. Instead, it appears to be a quite general and pervasive bias that characterizes people of all ages, not just adolescents (Fischhoff and Quadrel 1991; Millstein and Halpern-Felsher 2002; Quadrel et al. 1993; Reyna and Farley 2006).

The relation between perceived vulnerability and health-risk behaviors is unclear. Some research indicates that adolescents who are engaged in risky behavior such as smoking (Milam et al. 2000), drinking (Cohn et al. 1995), and high-risk sex (Murphy et al. 1998) are aware of the heightened risk but engage in those behaviors anyway (Reyna and Farley 2006). At the same time, other studies indicate that individuals engaged in risky behavior underestimate the risk, as would be predicted by rational models of behavior like the health-belief model (Reyna and Farley 2006). Consistent with this, low health literacy is associated with greater general risk-taking behavior in adolescents (DeWalt and Hink 2009).

It may be that these conflicting findings reflect the behavior of different types of risk-takers; alternately, among youth engaging in risky behavior, some may have or observe negative outcomes whereas others may not, leading to different risk perceptions over time. There is evidence that risk perceptions are highest among younger adolescents, and that older youth who have engaged in risky behavior without significant consequences may downgrade their risk perceptions accordingly (Halpern-Felsher et al. 2001; Reyna and Farley 2006). For youth with chronic illness, this would argue against allowing them too much freedom to "learn from their mistakes" (Sawyer and Aroni 2005), as they might instead learn that the odds of something bad happening *from any single behavior* are relatively low, although the combined odds approach certainty when they engage in behavior recurrently (Reyna and Farley 2006). In support of this, data suggest that when adolescents have positive experiences with behaviors such as drinking alcohol they are more likely to engage in that behavior in the future (Goldberg et al. 2002).

Clinical implications of the cognitive findings The findings presented above lead to a counter-intuitive conclusion. If youth tend to weigh potential costs against the benefits of engaging in risky behaviors, then presenting them with more factual information about risk can actually backfire. As noted above, teens overestimate many risks (Millstein and Halpern-Felsher 2002; Reyna and Adam 2003), so presenting them with more accurate information might lead them to think that the risk is not so high after all.

Consider a recent brochure about marijuana aimed at teens titled "Drugs: Shatter the Myths" (NIH Publication No. 13-7589, 2013) which begins with the question, "Is marijuana addictive?" It then answers: "Yes. The chances of becoming addicted to marijuana or any drug are different for each person. For marijuana, around 1 in 11 people who use it become addicted. Could you be that one?" Reyna's research suggests that many adolescents would take 1 in 11 as good odds, and be *more* likely to smoke marijuana after reading this brochure, rather than less. (Better is a later page on nicotine, which presents the simple fact: "Most people who start smoking in their teens become regular smokers before they're 18.").

Indeed, there is now good evidence that educational programs that stress risk to teens don't work, and in some cases they cause harm. For example, studies of Drug Abuse and Resistance Education (DARE) Programs have shown either null results or iatrogenic effects, with participating children sometimes showing an increase in alcohol and drug use (Lilienfeld 2007).

Of course, adolescents do need to be provided with appropriate information about health risks and benefits. The work of Reyna and her colleagues suggests that this information should not be presented in terms of relative odds, which reinforces teens' tendency to weigh relative risks and benefits, but in terms of underlying gist. As noted by Reyna and Rivers (2008), Gibbons and Gerrard (1997) reach a similar conclusion via a different route. They argue that most health-risk behaviors have images associated with them (a classic example being the Marlboro Man), that these images are highly accessible, and that they influence teens' behavior. Specifically, the more favorable the image, the likelier it will be that a youth will engage in that behavior (Gibbons et al. 2003). This model has substantial empirical support

(Gerrard et al. 2008). Based on these and related findings, Reyna and Rivers (2008) suggest that an important, empirically-supported way to reduce teen risk is to "encourage the development of positive prototypes (gists) or images of healthy behaviors and negative images of unhealthy behaviors using visual depictions, films, novels, serial dramas and other emotionally evocative media."

It should be noted that is possible for images to backfire, especially if they focus solely on risks to the exclusion of benefits. Pictorial warnings about the dangerous of smoking are the paradigmatic example. There is some evidence that graphic, fear-inducing pictures of the negative effects of smoking can result in avoidance of the message or in "psychological reactance" (Brehm 1966), a motivational state in which a person reacts against a message to preserve a sense of freedom and autonomy (see, for example, Erceg-Hurn and Steed 2011). However, the majority of studies show that even extremely graphic negative images are powerful motivators for change among youth as well as adult (Hammond 2011).

Stress and Adherence

In addition to all of the changes described above, adolescence is also characterized by greatly increased levels of stress. Limbic system structures (amygdala in particular) involved in the over-reactivity of the social-emotional reward system are also implicated in heightened stress reactivity (Casey et al. 2010), and it has been suggested that stress may increase reward sensitivity by its effects on the dopamine system (Mather and Lighthall 2012). Chronic stress may also impair the ability of the prefrontal cortex to modulate limbic system reactivity (Garner 2013).

Stress in turn is associated with worse decision-making, as reviewed by Galván and Rahdar (2013). For example, excessive stress can result in hurried choices; there is also evidence that stress "exacerbates behavioral biases" to be either risk-seeking or risk-averse (Galván and Rahdar 2013). As youth are generally more risk-seeking (compared to children or adults), stress may heighten this trend.

In terms of health-risk behaviors, there is a clear and strong association between high levels of stress and behaviors such as alcohol, drug, and cigarette use (National Survey of American Attitudes on Substance Abuse VIII: Teens and Parents, 2003). Garner (2013) has suggested that many health-risk behaviors may be engaged in as ways to manage chronic stress, in particular by reducing (or "turning off") an overactive stress response, which has been termed "behavioral allostasis." Moreover, stressed youth may have greater difficulty delaying gratification (Fields et al. 2009).

Managing a chronic illness in the face of chronic stress can be exceptionally challenging. In addition to its effects on decision-making, delay gratification, and behavioral allostasis, stress causes increases in blood sugars, complicating illness management for youth with diabetes, and is associated with hypertension and obesity (Garner 2013). High stress levels are also more likely among minorities and impoverished families (Galván and Rahdar 2013), further adding to the risk faced by these most vulnerable families (Anderson 2012).

Changes in Parenting and Social Support

At the same time as the drive for novelty-seeking and reward-seeking behavior spikes, and the maturity gap is at its widest, and stress reaches new heights, parents begin to reduce the amount of oversight and supervision they provide (Laird et al. 2003). Many families struggle to find the right balance between oversight and autonomy support, and the transition can be bumpy, but it generally proceeds without calamity (Laursen and Collins 2009). For youth with chronic illness, the reduction of parental supervision contributes significantly to risk for declining illness control (see Chaps. 7 and 10).

As youth spend less time under parental supervision, they spend more time with friends (Larson and Verma 1999). In adults, social support is strongly associated with better adherence and illness control (DiMatteo 2004). In youth, findings regarding social support have generally been mixed, although peer conflict consistently predicts worse adherence and illness control. Palladino and Helgeson (2012) concluded from their review of qualitative studies of youth with type 1 diabetes that they "consider peers to have influence on [teens'] self-care behavior, but it is not clear whether this influence is positive or negative."

Another implication of the neurodevelopmental findings reviewed above is that peer support may not always be a good thing for a teen's chronic illness management. Youth with active social lives are likely to be faced with more temptations and opportunities to engage in risky behavior. Importantly, for youth with chronic illness, the risk does not have to come from the high risk behaviors most parents worry about (e.g., drugs, violence) or from peers who engage in such behaviors— simply going camping or going to MacDonald's with friends can create risk for teens who have to manage a chronic illness.

At the same time, interacting with peers who are engaged in risky behavior does pose additional risk to youth with chronic illness. It has long been thought that having an illness would protect youth against transitionally risky behavior, but this does not appear to be the case. In fact, some health-risk behaviors (smoking, alcohol abuse) may be *more* likely in youth with chronic illness, despite the even greater health risks they face as a result (Sawyer et al. 2007).

Summary and Conclusions

The studies reviewed in this chapter demonstrate that risk-taking behavior increases substantially in adolescence, the result of a combustible combination of normal neurodevelopment and greater freedom from parental control. We in turn have argued that nonadherence can be seen either as a risk-taking behavior itself, or as the result of the neurodevelopmental and social changes that underlie adolescent risk-taking.

Risk-taking, as suggested by Steinberg (2010) is normative in adolescence. It is biologically-driven and has adaptive features, leading youth to be open to new experiences and explore what the world has in store for them. At the same time, risk-taking is the leading cause of youth morbidity and mortality. Its primary character-istic is a heightened responsivity to reward, leading to a preference for short-term reward over long-term gain. This is not a recipe for good adherence to a medical regimen, which frequently "demands effort and sacrifice for long term goal without any apparent immediate benefit to the patient" (Wolpert and Anderson, 2001).

Adolescents, their parents, and their healthcare providers are all faced with ex-ceptional complexities when trying to manage a chronic illness. Current research findings converge on a picture of adolescence that is characterized by:

- Worse adherence and worse illness control
- Increased risk-taking behavior
- Dramatic changes in the body and brain
- Heightened reactivity to reward (especially immediate reward) and to social and emotion input
- Immature cognitive control
- Decreased parent involvement
- A tendency to weigh risks against benefits
- High levels of stress

No wonder adherence is worse in adolescence than at any other time!

Younger adolescents tend to see themselves as especially vulnerable (Reyna and Farley 2006). They are also more prone to peer conformity, which peaks around age 10 or 11 and declines thereafter (Steinberg and Monahan 2007). Middle ado-lescence is the time when the "maturity gap" between social-emotional reactivity and cognitive control is at its widest, and there is independent evidence that the tendency to favor risky choice also peaks at this age (Burnett et al. 2010). However, late adolescence still remains the time of greatest actual risk, primarily as a func-tion of increased opportunity for risk-taking, ability to drive (car accidents being the leading cause of death in teens; Kann et al. 2014), and greatly reduced (if not absent) monitoring by parents.

Older adolescents may have decreased perception of risk because they have ex-perience engaging in risk without negative consequences (Reyna and Farley 2006), but they are also beginning to shift to a more gist-based mode of reasoning, which should be somewhat protective. It is interesting to speculate that the development of the default network, which is known to be involved in some way in mentalizing and imagery, may contribute to the greater use of gist in determining whether a risky behavior "is worth it." Recent research also suggests that from early to late adolescence there is a developmental shift from more reactive to more reasoned processing (Pomery et al. 2009), presumably as the social-emotional system begins to "cool down" and cognitive control mechanisms exert greater force.

Many of the problematic health-risk behaviors begun in adolescence persist into adulthood, where they continue to wreak havoc on the population's health. A similar pattern is evident for nonadherence behaviors, which also tend to have their start in adolescence and, once established, can persist into adulthood. Thus, adolescence is both a time of greatly enhanced risk, but also of real opportunity, as interventions in adolescence can help prevent the decline of illness management and set the stage for more successful adherence in adulthood.

References

Adams CD, Dreyer ML, Dinakar C, Portnoy JM. Pediatric asthma: a look at adherence from the patient and family perspective. Curr Allergy Asthma Rep. 2004;4(6):425–32.

American Diabetes Association. Standards of medical care in diabetes—2014. Diabetes C. 2014;37(1):S14–80.

Amiel SA, Sherwin RS, Simonson DC, Lauritano AA, Tamborlane WV. Impaired insulin action in puberty: A contributing factor to poor glycemic control in adolescent with diabetes. NEJM. 1986;315:215–9.

Anderson BJ. Who forgot? the challenges of family responsibility for adherence in vulnerable pediatric populations. Pediatrics. 2012;129.5:e1324–5.

Arnett P. Emerging adulthood: the winding road from late teens through the twenties. New York: Oxford University Press; 2004.

Baird A, Fugelsang J, Bennett C. What were you thinking: an fMRI study of adolescent decision-making. New York, USA: Poster presented at Cognitive Neuroscience Society meeting; 2005 Apr 2005.

Bender BG. Risk-taking, depression, adherence, and symptom control in adolescents and young adults with asthma. Am J Respir Crit Care Med. 2006;173:953–7.

Bender BG, Klinnert MD. Psychological correlates of asthma severity and treatment outcome in children. In: Kotses H, Harver A, Editors. Self-management of asthma. New York: Marcel Dekker; 1998. pp. 63–88.

Bernheim A, Halfon O, Boutrel B. Controversies about the enhanced vulnerability of the adolescent brain to develop addiction. Front Pharmacol. 2013;4:4–118.

Berns GS, Moore S, Capra CM. Adolescent engagement in dangerous behaviors is associated with increased white matter maturity of frontal cortex. PLoS ONE. 2009;4(8):e6773.

Blakemore SJ. Imaging brain development: the adolescent brain. Neuroimage. 2012;61:397–406.

Blakemore SJ, Choudhury S. Development of the adolescent brain: implications for executive function and social cognition. J Child Psychol Psychiatry. 2006;47(3):296–312.

Blakemore S-J, Robbins TW. Decision-making in the adolescent brain. Nat Neurosci. 2012;15:1184–91.

Brehm JW. A theory of psychological reactance. New York: Academic Press; 1966.

Broyd SJ, Demanuele C, Debener S, Helps SK, James CJ, Sonuga-Barke EJS. Default-mode brain dysfunction in mental disorders: a systematic review. Neurosci Biobehav Rev. 2009;33(3):279–96.

Buckner RL, Snyder AZ, Shannon BJ, et al. Molecular, structural, and functional characterization of Alzheimer's disease: evidence for a relationship between default activity, amyloid, and memory. J Neurosci. 2005;25:7709–17.

Burnett S, Bault N, Coricelli G, Blakemore S. Adolescents' heightened risk-seeking in a probabilistic gambling task. Cogn Dev. 2010;25:183–96.

Carey S. Conceptual differences between children and adults. Mind Lang. 1988;3:167–81.

Casey BJ, Getz S, Galvan A. The adolescent brain. Dev Rev. 2008;28(1):62–77.

Casey BJ, Jones RM, Levita L, Libby V, Pattwell S, Ruberry S, Soliman F, Somerville LH. The storm and stress of adolescence: Insights from human imaging and mouse genetics. Dev Psychobiol. 2010;52(3):225–35.

Cohen B. Is expected utility theory normative for medical decision making? Med Decis Mak. 1996;16:1–6.

Cohn LD, Macfarlane S, Yanez C, Imai WK. Risk-perception: differences between adolescents and adults. Health Psychol. 1995;14:217–22.

Colver A, Longwell S. New understanding of adolescent brain development: relevance to transitional healthcare for young people with long term conditions. Arch Dis Child. 2013;98:902–7.

DeWalt DA, Hink A. Health literacy and child health outcomes: a systematic review of the literature. Pediatrics. 2009;124:S265–74.

DiMatteo MR. Social support and patient adherence to medical treatment: a meta-analysis. Health Psychol. 2004;23:207.

DiMatteo MR, Haskard KB, Williams SL. Health beliefs, disease severity, and patient adherence: a meta-analysis. Med Care. 2007;45:521–8.

Donovan JL. Patient decision making: the missing ingredient in compliance research. International journal of technology assessment in health care 1995; 11: 443–455.

Duke DC, Harris MA. Executive function, adherence, and glycemic control in adolescents with type 1 diabetes: a literature review. Curr Diab Rep. 2014 Oct;14(10):532.

Elkin TD, Whelan JP, Meyers AW, Phipps S, Glaser RR. The effect of achievement orientation on responses to success and failure in pediatric cancer patients. J Pediatric Psychol. 1998;23:67–76.

Erceg-Hurn DM, Steed LG. Does exposure to cigarette health warnings elicit psychological reactance in smokers? J Appl Soc Psychol. 2011;41(1):219–37.

Ernst M, Nelson E, Jazbec S, McClure E, Monk C, Blair R, Leibenluft E, Blair J, Pine D. Amygdala and nucleus accumbens activation in response to receipt and omission of gains in adults and adolescents. Neuroimage. 2005;25:1279–1291.

Fair DA, Cohen AL, Dosenbach NUF, Church JA, Miezin FM, Barch DM, Raichle ME, Petersen SE, Schlaggar BL. The maturing architecture of the brain's default network. Proc Natl Acad Sci USA. 2008;105:1028–32.

Fields S, Leraas K, Collins C, Reynolds B. Delay discounting as a mediator of the relationship between stress and cigarette smoking status in adolescents. Behav Pharmacol. 2009;20:455–60.

Fischhoff B, Quadrel M. Adolescent alcohol decisions. Alcohol Health and Research World 1991; 15: 43–51.

Galván A, Rahdar A. The neurobiological effects of stress on adolescent decision making. Neuroscience. 2013;249:223–31.

Galván A, Hare TA, Parra CE, Penn J, Voss H, Glover G, Casey BJ. Earlier development of the accumbens relative to orbitalfrontal cortex might underlie risk-taking behavior in adolescence. J Neurosci. 2006;26:6885–92.

Gardner M, Steinberg L. Peer influence on risk taking, risk preference, and risky decision making in adolescence and adulthood: an experimental study. Dev Psychol. 2005;41:625–35.

Garner AS. Home visiting and the biology of toxic stress: opportunities to address early childhood adversity. Pediatrics. 2013;132:S6.

Gerrard M, Gibbons FX, Gano M. Adolescents' risk perceptions and behavioral willingness: implications for intervention. In: Romer D, Editor. Reducing adolescent risk: toward an integrated approach. Thousand Oaks: Sage; 2003. pp. 75–82.

Gerrard M, Gibbons FX, Houlihan AE, Stock ML, Pomery EA. A dual-process approach to health risk decision-making: the prototype-willingness model. Dev Rev. 2008;28:29–61.

Gibbons FX. Intention, expectation, and willingness 2008. http://cancercontrol.cancer.gov/BRP/constructs/intent-expect-willingness/iew4.html.

Gibbons FX, Gerrard M. Health images and their effects on health behavior. In: Buunk BP, Gibbons FX, Editors. Health, coping, and well-being: perspectives from social comparison theory. Mahwah: Lawrence Erlbaum Associates; 1997. pp. 63–94.

Gibbons FX, Gerrard M, Blanton H, Russell DW. Reasoned action and social reaction: willingness and intention as independent predictors of health risk. J Pers Soc Psychol. 1998a;74(5):1164.

Gibbons FX, Gerrard M, Lane DJ. A social reaction model of adolescent health risk. In: Suls J, Wallston KA, Editors. Social psychological foundations of health and illness. Blackwell series in health psychology and behavioral medicine. Malden: Blackwell; 2003. pp. 107–36.

Gibbons FX, Gerrard M, Vande Lune LS, Wills TA, Brody G, Conger RD. Context and cognition: environmental risk, social influence, and adolescent substance use. Pers Soc Psychol Bull. 2004;30:1048–61.

Gibbons FX, Gerrard M, Reimer RA, Pomery EA. Unintentional behavior: a subrational approach to health risk. In: de Ridder D, de Wit J, Editors. New perspectives on health behavior: The role of self-regulation. Chichester: Wiley; 2005.

Gibbons FX, Gerrard M, McCaul KD, editors. Constructs and measures web resource. National Cancer Institute Internet Web Site; 2006. [Retrieved 3/15/2015]. Behavioral intentions, expectations, and willingness. http://cancercontrol.cancer.gov/brp/constructs/intent-expect-willingness/index.html.

Giedd JN. The teen brain: Insights from neuroimaging. J Adolesc Health. 2008;42:335–43.

Goldberg JH, Halpern-Felsher BL, Millstein SG. Beyond invulnerability: the importance of benefits in adolescents' decision to drink alcohol. Health Psychol. 2002;21:477–84.

Halpern-Felsher BL, Millstein SG, Ellen JM, Adler NE, Tschann JM, Biehl M. The role of behavioral experience in judging risks. Health Psychol. 2001; 20(2):120–6.

Hammond D. Health warning messages on tobacco products: a review. Tob Control. 2011;20:e327–37.

Helgeson VS, Siminerio L, Escobar O, Becker D. Predictors of metabolic control among adolescents with diabetes: a 4-year longitudinal study. J Pediatr Psychol. 2009;34:254–70.

Hilliard JP, Fritz GF, Lewiston NJ. Levels of aspiration of parents for their asthmatic, diabetic, and healthy children. J Clin Psychol. 1985;41:587–97.

Horne R, Weinman I. Patients' beliefs about prescribed medicines and their role in adherence to treatment in chronic physical illness. Psychosom Res. 1999;47:555–67. Janz NK, Becker MH. The health belief model: a decade later. Health Educ Behav. 1984;11(1):1–47.

Kann L, Steve K, Shari LS, Katherine HF, Joseph K, William AH, Richard L, et al. "Youth risk behavior surveillance-United States, 2013." MMWR: Surveillance Summaries 63, no. SS-04 2014:1–168.

Kaufmann L, Pixner S, Starke M, et al. Neurocognition and brain structure in pediatric patients with type 1 diabetes. J Pediatr Neuroradiol. 2011: Neurocognition and brain structure in pediatric patients with type 1 diabetes.

Kessler RC, Berglund P, Delmer O, Jin R, Merikangas KR, Walters EE. Lifetime prevalence and age-of-onset distributions of DSM-IV disorders in the National Comorbidity Survey Replication. Arch Gen Psychiatry. 2005;62:593–602.

Kondryn et al. 2011, Taddeo D, Egedy M, Frappier J-Y. Adherence to treatment in adolescents. Paediatr Child Health. 2008;13(1):19–24.

Kovacs M, Goldston D, Obrosky S, Iyengar S. Prevalence and predictors of pervasive non-compliance with medical treatment among youths with insulin-dependent diabetes mellitus. J Am Acad Child Adol Psychiatry. 1992;31:1112–9.

Laird RD, Pettit GS, Bates JE, Dodge KA. Parents' monitoring-relevant knowledge and adolescents' delinquent behavior: Evidence of correlated developmental changes and reciprocal influences. Child Dev. 2003;74:752–68.

Larson RW, Verma S. How children and adolescents spend time across the world: Work, play, and developmental opportunities. Psychol Bull. 1999;125(6):701–36.

Laursen B, Collins WA. Parent–adolescent relationships during adolescence. In: Lerner RM, Steinberg L, Editors. Handbook of adolescent psychology. 3rd edn. Vol. 2. Hoboken: Wiley; 2009. pp. 3–42.

Lenroot RK, Giedd JN. Brain development in children and adolescents: insights from anatomical magnetic resonance imaging. Neurosci Biobehav Rev. 2006;30:718–29.

Lilienfeld SO. Psychological treatments that cause harm perspectives on psychological science 2007.

Luna B, Padmanabhan A, O'Hearn K. What has fMRI told us about the development of cognitive control through adolescence? Brain Cogn. 2010;72:101–13. doi:10.1016/j.bandc.2009.08.005.

Mather M, Lighthall N. Both risk and reward are processed differently in decisions made under stress. Curr Dir Psychol Sci. 2012;21:36–41.

McClure SM, Laibson DI, Lowenstein G, Cohen JD. Separate neural systems value immediate and delayed monetary rewards. Science. 2004;306:503–7.

Metcalfe J, Mischel W. A hot/cool-system analysis of delay of gratification: dynamics of willpower. Psychol Rev. 1999;106:3–19.

Milam JE, Sussman S, Ritt-Olson A, Dent CW. Perceived invulnerability and cigarette smoking among adolescents. Addict Behav. 2000 Jan–Feb;25(1):71–80.

Millstein SG, Halpern-Felsher BL. Judgments about risk and perceived invulnerability in adolescents and young adults. J Res Adolesc. 2002;12:399–422.

Murphy DA, Rotheram-Borus MJ, Reid HM. Adolescent gender differences in HIV-related sexual risk acts, social-cognitive, factors and behavioral skills. J Adolesc. 1998;21:197–20.

National Survey of American Attitudes on Substance Abuse VIII. Teens and Parents. 2003; New York: National Center on Addiction and Substance Abuse at Columbia University.

NIH Publication No. 13–7589. 2013. http://drugfactsweek.drugabuse.gov/files/teenbrochure_508. pdf. Accessed 15 Mar 2015.

Olson E, Collins P, Hooper C, Muetzel R, Lim K, Luciana M. White matter integrity predicts delay discounting behavior in 9- to 23-year-olds: a diffusion tensor imaging study. J Cognit Neurosci. 2008;21:1406–21.

Palladino DK, Vicki SH. Friends or foes? a review of peer influence on self-care and glycemic control in adolescents with type 1 diabetes. J Pediatric Psychol. 2012;37(5):591–603.

Patino AM, Sanchez J, Eidson M, Delamater AM. Health beliefs and regimen adherence in minority adolescents with type 1 diabetes. J Pediatric Psychol. 2005;30(6):503–12.

Paus T, Zijdenbos A, Worsley K, Collins DL, Blumenthal J, Giedd JN, et al. Structural maturation of neural pathways in children and adolescents: in vivo study. Science. 1999;283:1908–11.

Perantie DC, Wu J, Koller JM, et al. Regional brain volume differences associated with hyperglycemia and severe hypoglycemia in youth with type 1 diabetes. Diabetes C. 2007;30:2331–7.

Pomery EA, Gibbons FX, Reis-Bergan M, Gerrard M. From willingness to intention: Experience moderates the shift from reactive to reasoned behavior. Pers Soc Psychol Bull. 2009 July;35(7):894–908.

Power JD, Fair DA, Schlaggar BL, Petersen SE. The development of human functional brain networks. Neuron. 2010;67(5):735–48.

Quadrel MJ, Fischhoff B, Davis W. Adolescent (in)vulnerability. American Psychologist, 1993; 48, 102–116.

Rapoff MA. Adherence to pediatric medical regimens (2nd ed.). New York: Springer; 2010.

Reyna VF. How people make decisions that involve risk: a dual process approach. Curr Dir Psychol Sci. 2004;13:60–6.

Reyna VF, Adam MB, Poirier K, LeCroy CW, Brainerd CJ. Risky decision-making in childhood and adolescence: a fuzzy-trace theory approach. In: Jacobs J, Klacynski P, Editors. The development of judgment and decision-making in children and adolescents. Mahwah: Erlbaum; 2005. pp. 77–106.

Reyna VF, Adam MB. Fuzzy-trace theory, risk communication, and product labeling in sexually transmitted diseases. Risk Anal. 2003;23:325–42.

Reyna VF, Farley F. Risk and rationality in adolescent decision-making: Implications for theory, practice, and public policy. Psychol Sci Pub Interest. 2006;7:1–44.

Reyna VF, Rivers SE. Current theories of risk and rational decision making. Dev Rev. 2008;28(1):1–11.

Sawyer SM, Aroni RA. Self-management in adolescents with chronic illness. What does it mean and how can it be achieved? Med J Aust. 2005 Oct 17;183(8):405–9.

Sawyer SM, Drew S, Yeo MS. Adolescents with a chronic condition: challenges living, challenges treating. Lancet. 2007;369:(9571)1481–9.

Schwartz DD, Wasserman R, Powell PW, Axelrad ME. Neurocognitive outcomes in pediatric diabetes: a developmental perspective. Curr Diabetes Rep. 2014;10:533.

Seiffge-Krenke I. Chronic disease and perceived developmental progression in adolescence. Dev Psychol. 1998;34:1073–84.

Steinberg L. A social neuroscience perspective on adolescent risk-taking. Dev Rev. 2008;28:78–106.

Steinberg L. A behavioral scientist looks at the science of adolescent brain development. Brain Cogn. 2010;72:160–4.

Steinberg L. Should the science of adolescent brain development inform public policy? Lecture delivered at the National Academy of Sciences on November 3, 2011. http://issues.org/28-3/steinberg/. Accessed 15 Mar 2015.

Steinberg L, Monahan KC. Age differences in resistance to peer influence. Dev Psychol. 2007;43(6):1531–43.

Supekar K, Uddin LQ, Prater K, Amin H, Greicius MD, Menon V. Development of functional and structural connectivity within the default mode network in young children. NeuroImage. 2010;52(1):290–301.

Taddeo D, Egedy M, Frappier JY. Adherence to treatment in adolescents. Paediatr Child Health. 2008;13:19–24.

Wolpert HA, Anderson BJ. Management of diabetes: are doctors framing the benefits from the wrong perspective? BMJ. 2001;323:994–6.

Yurgelun-Todd D. Emotional and cognitive changes during adolescence. Curr Opin Neurobiol. 2007;17:251–7.

Chapter 7
The Role of Parents

In contrast to warnings about the dangers of over-parenting, the child development literature is replete with evidence that parental involvement in children's lives facilitates healthy development.... On the other hand, some research has suggested that too much parental involvement may lead to negative child outcomes.

—Schiffrin et al. 2013

Abstract Having a child with a chronic illness places a substantial burden on parents. In early and middle childhood, the parent must shoulder complete responsibility for illness management; as the child enters adolescence, responsibility begins to be shared, and parenting gradually shifts from efforts to gain child compliance to efforts to support the youth's increasing autonomy. This is a delicate dance, often fraught with the danger of descending into a cycle of parent-child conflict. Yet the research literature is very clear—maintaining positive parent involvement from childhood through even late adolescence is strongly associated with better adherence, better illness control, and better child quality of life. how to maintain involvement in a positive way without devolving into conflict is the focus of this chapter. We discuss important aspects of effective, positive parenting, and the ways parenting can go wrong despite only intending to do well.

In the preceding chapters we discussed the challenges and complexities in managing a child's chronic illness. A point that may have been lost is that adherence problems are not specific to children and adolescents—in fact, estimated rates of nonadherence in adult populations are comparable (Sabate 2003). Yet children, often as young as 12 or even 10, are given primary responsibility for managing their illness. As we noted earlier, if adults struggle so much with adherence, how can we expect children to do better?

The answer, of course, is that they can't. Fortunately, most children can benefit from the involvement of one or more concerned adults in managing their illness. When done right, parent support is one of the strongest predictors of successful health outcomes in children with diabetes, and parent disengagement or parent-

© Springer International Publishing Switzerland 2015

D. D. Schwartz, M. E. Axelrad, *Healthcare Partnerships for Pediatric Adherence,*
SpringerBriefs in Public Health, DOI 10.1007/978-3-319-13668-4_7

child conflict are some of the strongest predictors of problematic adherence and poor illness control (Delamater et al. 2001).

Parent Involvement

Children with involved parents tend to fare better across almost all areas of development—academically, emotionally, behaviorally, and socially (Schiffrin et al. 2013)—whereas the converse is also true: children with uninvolved parents tend to do worse (e.g., Pomerantz et al. 2007). The National Longitudinal Study of Adolescent Health (Resnick et al. 1997) found that parent involvement in adolescence was the strongest predictor of risky behavior such as substance use and unprotected sex.

The same patterns hold for children with chronic illness. When parent involvement decreases, and children take on primary responsibility for illness management, adherence and illness control can suffer (Kahana et al. 2008; Chaps. 7 and 10). Reduced parent involvement/lack of monitoring is also associated with increased risk for serious acute complications such as DKA in diabetes patients and organ transplant loss. Other research suggests that adolescents' *perception* of parent involvement is also important, with greater perceived involvement (especially around coping with stress) being associated with better adherence (Wiebe et al. 2005).

However, as noted by many authors, not all involvement is equal. Research indicates that certain aspects of parenting and parent involvement are actually associated with worse outcomes. This occurs when parents' involvement is perceived as overly controlling, intrusive, or negative (Schiffrin et al. 2013; Seiffge-Krenke et al. 2013; Wiebe et al. 2005), or conflict results (Hood et al. 2007). In such circumstances, adherence can suffer. In the words of Weissberg-Benchell et al. (2009), "the manner in which parents demonstrate involvement in diabetes management is more important than the specific amount of responsibility taken by the parent."

Parenting Styles

The classic contemporary model of parenting, developed by Diana Baumrind (1971), identified two dimensions of parenting (control versus warmth/acceptance) that in turn yield four different parenting styles.

- *Authoritative* parents are high in both dimensions. They provide significant structure and limit-setting in a context of parental warmth.
- *Authoritarian* parents are high in control but low in warmth. They tend to be more punitive, negative, and critical. Authoritarian parents may receive immediate compliance, but at the cost of increased parent-child conflict and decreased behavioral compliance over time.

- *Permissive* parents are low in control but high in warmth. They give their children a lot of freedom and support, and are reluctant to set limits. Permissive parents make few demands on their children, making it difficult for the child to learn to regulate his behavior and consistently follow routines, including routines involved in illness management.
- *Uninvolved* parents are low in both dimensions. They allow their children a significant amount of freedom but may seem (or be) disinterested in the outcome.

In general, authoritative parenting has been associated with the best outcomes, both in terms of general development and child functioning (Barber et al. 2005), and with regards to adherence and chronic illness control both in younger children (e.g., Davis et al. 2001; Monaghan et al. 2012) and adolescents (e.g., Shorer et al. 2011). Parental *warmth, support, and acceptance* (all aspects of authoritative parenting) are incontrovertibly associated with positive child outcomes in almost every area examined, and at any age, and this includes adherence (Butler et al. 2007; Davis et al. 2001; Monaghan et al. 2012). In contrast, parenting that is overly negative and critical (Armstrong and Streisand 2011) is strongly associated with worse psychological outcomes, lower adherence, and worse illness control.

The results for *parental control* are more complicated, depending on the developmental stage of the child (Butler et al. 2007), how control is defined, and especially how it is perceived (Wiebe et al. 2005).

Parental Control

Positive aspects of parent control include providing appropriate limits and monitoring children's and youth's behaviors, both to ensure that adherence behaviors get done and that risk-taking behaviors are minimized. However, parents can attempt to exert too much control, giving their children little say and limiting them even from developmentally appropriate activities Overly controlling behavior has been associated with increased behavior problems among children, although whether this is cause or effect or an interaction has been debated—for example, parents may become more controlling in response to child behavior problems, as an attempt to reign the behaviors in, or children may escalate their behavior in the face of parent control, as a way of asserting their own autonomy.

Two types of parental control have been distinguished in the literature: behavioral control and psychological control. These types of control have been shown to have very different effects on child outcomes.

Behavioral control, which involves parental monitoring and limit-setting, and is seen as being oriented toward socialization and behavioral regulation (Silk et al. 2003). Parental behavioral control has generally been shown to be associated with positive child outcomes (Barber et al. 1994), although it may begin to have negative effects when youth reach early adulthood (Helgeson et al. 2014; Schiffrin et al. 2013). Surprisingly, most studies examining behavioral control on chronic illness outcomes have found negative effects (Butler et al. 2007; Davis et al. 2001; Wiebe et al. 2005), although this probably has to do with control was operationalized in these studies (e.g., Weibe et al.: "mother told the child what to do or was too involved"; Butler et al.: parent "insists that you must do exactly as you are told"; Helgeson et al.: "Do you feel as though your parents control everything in your life?" "Do you feel that your parents demand to know everything?"). These constructs of "excessive firm control" or "strictness" differ from the sort of limit-setting typically associated with the authoritative parenting style. Parental monitoring, arguably a less excessive form of limit-setting, has consistently been found to be associated with better regimen adherence (e.g., Ellis et al. 2007).

Psychological control involves manipulative parent behaviors focused on using guilt, shame, and contingent love and acceptance to pressure a child into conforming with parent expectations (Barber 1996), or efforts to control the child's thoughts and feelings (Butler et al. 2007). In contrast to behavioral control, psychologically controlling behavior has consistently been found to be detrimental to children's general well-being (e.g., Barber et al. 2005). Studies have supported the negative effects of psychological control on chronic illness outcomes as well (e.g., Weissberg-Benchell et al. 2009).

There is also evidence that parental control may have different effects for children with and without a chronic illness. A recent study by Helgeson and colleagues (2014) examined whether perceptions of parent support and control in early adolescence were predictive of risk behavior and health outcomes in emerging adulthood in youth with and without type 1 diabetes. Consistent with other studies, they found that excessive parent control was associated with a range of negative outcomes, including increased risk for smoking and reduced likelihood of attending college. Excessive control also predicted increased risk for depression in youth without diabetes. However, in youth with diabetes, the results were dramatically different. Parental controlling behavior in adolescence was associated with reduced risk for depressive symptoms and clinical depression in emerging adults with diabetes, and better diabetes self-care.

Why would parent control have such different effects for youth with and without a chronic illness? Helgeson et al. note the importance of parent involvement for good illness care, and speculate that for youth with diabetes (and presumably other chronic illnesses), "parent controlling behavior may reflect parent involvement." The implication is that youth with chronic illness "may expect a higher level of parental involvement than other youth and be more likely to construe a lack of parental control as a lack of involvement in their lives." Thus, parent behaviors that may seem overly controlling to many youth might instead be seen as necessary guidance and input by youth burdened with a chronic illness.

Of course, control is also somewhat in the eye of the beholder: what one person perceives as controlling, another will view as necessary support (Wiebe et al. 2005). Other factors such as the parent's positive or negative affect, warmth, and communication style likely influence whether involvement is perceived as supportive or controlling. When involvement is coupled with criticism, for example, an adolescent may be made to feel incompetent (Pomerantz and Eaton 2000), reducing her sense of self-efficacy and her motivation to participate in her care (Wiebe et al. 2005). When parent involvement is coupled with negative affect, a pattern of parent-child conflict may also result.

The Transactional Nature of Parenting

It should also be kept in mind that parenting is often a *response* to child behaviors, and not necessarily the initial cause. For example, lower child engagement in school, which has been postulated to *result* from over-involved parenting (e.g., Padilla-Walker and Nelson 2012), may actually *precipitate* greater parent involvement and attempts at control.

In fact, this is a pattern we frequently see in families of children with a chronic illness. It often goes something like this: A 14 year-old with type 1 diabetes is given primary responsibility for illness management with little parent oversight. Over time, his adherence behaviors and metabolic control decline. When his mother discovers that his A1c has climbed to 10%, she steps back in and steps up her efforts to help, typically with some comments to the effect that she is disappointed and had expected her son to do better. Rather than accept her renewed involvement, however, the son tries to shut her out, sullenly saying he "can do this on his own." This concerns his mother, who begins to nag and cajole him to take better care of his diabetes, but this backfires further, as her son becomes more resistant to complying as a way to preserve his sense of freedom and control. This is a well-documented pattern that has been termed *miscarried helping*.

Miscarried Helping

Miscarried helping (Anderson and Coyne 1991; Coyne et al. 1988) refers to an interaction pattern parents can fall into with their children over chronic illness management, in which parental attempts to help the youth backfire because they are perceived as overly intrusive, coercive, or critical. Central to the phenomenon is parent worry and concern, which can make the interaction highly emotional for both parent and child. In response to the parent's efforts, the child becomes more resistant, and the parent steps up her efforts further; the result is a downward spiral of conflict that often ends in parent disengagement from care (Hafen and Laursen 2009; Kerr et al. 2008). Unfortunately this disengagement occurs just when more support is needed.

Miscarried helping is associated with worse adherence and poorer metabolic control in youth with type 1 diabetes, and it likely has similar effects in other illness groups (Drotar and Bonner 2009).

Racial/Ethnic Differences in Parenting

Discussions of parenting invariably raise questions about parenting differences between racial and ethnic groups, and whether research based on one group (typically middle class whites) is truly applicable to others. In general, the research appears to support the general benefits of authoritative parenting for African American youth (Steinberg et al. 1991), although involvement of fathers may play a particularly important role (Bean et al. 2006). Other research suggests that there may be a subgroup of African American parents who have a mixed style of parenting (a combination of strict and stern but emotionally warm control—what the authors called "tough love") that may be equally effective (Brooks-Gunn and Markman 2005).

Few studies have examined racial/ethnic differences in parenting and their relation to adherence or chronic illness control. In a study of children with type 1 diabetes (Davis et al. 2001), African American parents were significantly higher on strict control and their children had worse glycemic control, but parenting was not associated with glycemic control when race/ethnicity was entered in the analyses.

Parenting Stress

Unfortunately, parent involvement does not come without costs. Parents of children with a chronic illness are often at greater psychological risk than their children, and parental well-being and psychopathology are strongly associated with children's health outcomes and adherence (Kazak et al. 2012). For example, symptoms of post traumatic stress (although not the full disorder) are highly elevated in parents of children with cancer (Kazak et al. 1997), type 1 diabetes (Cline et al. 2011; Landolt et al. 2002), organ transplant (Young et al. 2003), and children admitted to a hospital PICU (Balluffi et al. 2004).

Parents (especially mothers) also tend to bear the brunt of illness management responsibility, and many endure significant conflict with their child as a result. A recent systematic review found significantly higher parenting stress among caregivers of children with asthma, cancer, cystic fibrosis, diabetes, epilepsy, juvenile rheumatoid arthritis, and sickle cell disease compared to caregivers of healthy children, with an overall effect size of 0.40 (Cousino and Hazen 2013), and that stress was directly associated with parents having greater responsibility for illness management. A child's nonadherent behavior is also a source of stress for many parents (Powers et al. 2002).

Parenting stress is associated with worse adherence in children with different medical conditions, including asthma (DeMore et al. 2005), and organ transplant (Gerson et al. 2004). Managing parenting stress is likely to be important to developing effective parent-child collaboration. Interestingly, authoritative parenting may help reduce pediatric parenting stress, possibly through its effects on child behavioral compliance and better adherence (Monaghan et al. 2012).

Positive Parenting Can Reduce Risk

As noted above, positive or authoritative parenting is associated with better psychosocial and behavioral outcomes for children. Importantly, these effects do not appear to be restricted to younger children. Studies suggest that positive parenting is associated with emotional- and self-regulation in teens, and may influence engagement in health-risk behaviors such as alcohol consumption (Brody and Ge 2001). Recent longitudinal research has also shown that positive parenting during conflict predicts reduced incidence of depressive disorders in teens years later (O.S. Schwartz et al. 2014).

Intriguingly, parenting may actually affect adolescent brain development. In another longitudinal investigation using structural MRI, Whittle et al. (2014) found that positive parenting in early adolescence was associated with advanced maturation of the amygdala, orbital frontal cortex, and anterior cingulated cortex in later adolescence. These brain areas are involved in reward processing, emotional reactivity, and emotional regulation, and they are some of the same areas also involved in risky behavior in teens, as discussed in Chap. 6. Thus, these finding suggest that positive parenting may affect self-regulation—and risk-taking behavior—through its direct effects on brain development.

As discussed in Chap. 8, positive parenting can also buffer children from the effects of toxic stress (National Scientific Council on the Developing Child 2004). In fact, it is seen as the single factor that can make potentially toxic stressors tolerable, and allow children to shut off the stress response before it becomes permanently dysregulated. The National Scientific Council on the Developing Child and the American Academy of Pediatrics both view the promotion of positive parenting as the cornerstone of efforts to reduce health disparities related to toxic stress (Garner et al. 2012).

These observations raise the interesting question of whether positive parenting might reduce the risk for nonadherence. Studies demonstrating the effectiveness of parenting teamwork interventions (e.g., Anderson et al 1999; Duncan et al. 2013) would suggest that the answer is yes. Parent training in positive parenting techniques at or around the time when a chronic illness is diagnosed might therefore help reduce the likelihood of the subsequent emergence of nonadherent behaviors, especially among higher risk families.

Evidence-Based Parenting Interventions

As noted by Garner et al. (2012), there are a number of evidence-based interventions that promote positive parenting, including Triple P, Incredible Years, Home visiting, and Nurturing Parenting. Triple P may be of special interest to pediatricians and other healthcare providers, as the program offers training in evidence-based approaches to working with parents to foster positive parenting and prevent behavioral or emotional problems in children, using a brief consultation model adapted for primary care settings (see http://www.triplep.net/glo-en/home/).

Summary and Conclusions

The research we have reviewed so far strongly supports the value and importance of continued parent involvement in chronic illness management. It has also revealed a pitfall of maintaining high levels of involvement in adolescence, in that involvement can backfire and result in feelings of inadequacy or in a pattern of coercive parenting and parent-child conflict, especially in adolescence. As discussed in Chap. 6, normal developmental changes in adolescence drive this interaction to some degree. At the same time, parenting style appears to mediate the relationship between parent involvement and either positive or negative outcomes. Specifically, outcomes are optimized when parent involvement is accompanied by other aspects of positive parenting and conflict is minimized. We return to these issues in Part II of this volume, where we argue that it is time to rethink the prevailing focus on pediatric self-management in favor of a more family-centered view.

References

Anderson BJ, Coyne JC. "Miscarried helping" in the interactions between chronically ill children and their parents. In: Johnson JH, Johnson SB, Editors. Advances in child health psychology. Gainesville: University of Florida Press; 1991. pp. 167–77.

Anderson B, Brackett J, Ho J, Laffel LM. An office-based intervention to maintain parent-adolescent teamwork in diabetes management. Impact on parent involvement, family conflict, and subsequent glycemic control. Diabetes C. 1999;22:713–21.

Armstrong B, Mackey ER, Streisand R. Parenting behavior, child functioning, and health behaviors in preadolescents with type 1 diabetes. J Pediatr Psychol 2011;36:1052–61.

Balluffi A, Kassam-Adams N, Kazak A, Tucker M, Dominguez T, Helfaer M. Traumatic stress in parents of children admitted to the pediatric intensive care unit. Pediatric Crit C Med. 2004;5(6):547–53.

Barber BK. Parental psychological control: revisiting a neglected construct. Child Dev. 1996;67:3296–319.

Barber BK, Olsen JE, Shagle SC. Associations between parental psychological and behavioral control and youth internalized and externalized behaviors. Child Dev. 1994;65:1120–36.

Barber BK, Stolz HE, Olsen JA. Parental support, psychological control, and behavioral control: assessing relevance across time, culture, and method. In: Overton WF, Editor. Monographs of the society for research in child development (Series 282, Vol. 70)Boston: Blackwell; 2005.

Baumrind D. Current patterns of parental authority. Developmental psychology monographs, 4 (1, Pt.2); [Baumrind, D. (1991). Effective parenting during the early adolescent transition]. In: Cowan PA, Hetherington EM, Editors. Advances in family research (Vol. 2). Hillsdale: Erlbaum; 1971.

Bean RA, Barber BK, Crane DR. Parental support, behavioral control, and psychological control among African American youth: the relationship to academic grades, delinquency, and depression. J Fam Issue. 2006;27:1335–55.

Brody GH, Ge XJ. Linking parenting processes and self-regulation to psychological functioning and alcohol use during early adolescence. J Fam Psychol. 2001;20(4):1014–43.

Brooks-Gunn J, Markman LB. The contribution of parenting to ethnic and racial gaps in school readiness. Future Child. 2005;15(1):139–68.

Butler JM, Skinner M, Gelfand D, Berg CA, Wiebe DJ. Maternal parenting style and adjustment in adolescents with type I diabetes. J Pediatr Psychol. 2007;32:1227–37.

Cline VD, Schwartz DD, Axelrad ME, Anderson BJ. A pilot study of acute stress symptoms in parents and youth following diagnosis of type I diabetes. J Clin Psychol Med Set. 2011;18:416–22.

Cousino MK, Hazen RA. Parenting stress among caregivers of children with chronic illness: a systematic review. J Pediatr Psychol. 2013;38:809–28.

Coyne JC, Wortman CB, Lehman DR. The other side of support: emotional overinvolvement and miscarried helping. In Gottlieb BH Editor. Marshalling Social Support: Formats, Processes, and Effects. Sage Publications: Newbury Park, 1988.

Davis CL, Delamater AM, Shaw KH, La Greca AM, Eidson MS, Perez-Rodriguez JE, Nemery R. Parenting styles, regimen adherence, and glycemic control in 4- to 10-year-old children with diabetes. J Pediatr Psychol. 2001;26:123–9. (Monaghan et al. 2012)

Delamater AM, Jacobson AM, Anderson B, Cox D, Fisher L, Lustman P, Rubin R, Wysocki T. Psychosocial therapies in diabetes report of the psychosocial therapies working group. Diabetes C. 2001;24:1286–92.

De More M, Adams C, Wilson N, Hogan MB. Parenting stress, difficult child behavior, and use of routines in relation to adherence in pediatric asthma. Child Health C. 2005;34:245–59.

Drotar D, Bonner MS. Influences on adherence to pediatric asthma treatment: a review of correlates and predictors. J Dev Behav Pediatrics. 2009;30:574–82.

Duncan CL, Hogan MB, Tien KJ, … Portnoy J. Efficacy of a parent-youth teamwork intervention to promote adherence in pediatric asthma. J Pediatr Psychol. 2013;38:617–28.

Ellis DA, Podolski C, Frey M, et al. The role of parental monitoring in adolescent health outcomes: Impact on regimen adherence in youth with type 1 diabetes. J Pediatr Psychol. 2007;32:907–17.

Garner AS, et al. Early childhood adversity, toxic stress, and the role of the pediatrician: translating developmental science into lifelong health. Pediatrics. 2012;129,e224–31.

Gerson AC, Furth SL, Neu AM, Fivush BA. Assessing associations between medication adherence and potentially modifiable psychosocial variables in pediatric kidney transplant recipients and their families. Pediatric Transplant. 2004;8:543–50.

Hafen CA, Laursen B. More problems and less support: early adolescent adjustment forecasts changes in perceived support from parents. J Fam Psychol. 2009;23:193–202.

Helgeson VS, Palladino DK, Reynolds KA, Becker D, Escobar O, Siminerio L. Early adolescent relationship predictors of emerging adult outcomes: youth with and without type 1 diabetes. Ann Behav Med. 2014;47(3):270–9.

Hood KK, Butler DA, Anderson BJ, Laffel LM. Updated and revised diabetes family conflict scale. Diabetes C. 2007;30:1764–9.

Kahana S, Drotar D, Frazier T. Meta-analysis of psychological interventions to promote adherence to treatment in pediatric chronic health conditions. J Pediatr Psychol. 2008;33:590–611.

Kazak AE, Anne E, Barakat LP, Meeske K, Christakis D, Meadows AT, Rosemary C, Biancamaria P, Margaret LS. Posttraumatic stress, family functioning, and social support in survivors of childhood leukemia and their mothers and fathers. J Consult Clin Psychol. 1997;65(1): 120.

Kazak AE, Brier M, Alderfer MA, Reilly A, Parker SF, Rogerwick S, Ditaranto S, Barakat LP. Screening for psychosocial risk in pediatric cancer. Pediatric Blood Cancer 2012;59:822–7.

Kerr M, Stattin H, Pakalniskiene V. Parents react to adolescent problem behaviors by worrying more and monitoring less. In: Kerr M, Stattin H, Engels RCME, Editors. What can parents do? New insights into the role of parents in adolescent problem behavior. New York: Wiley; 2008. pp. 91–112.

Landolt MA, Ribi K, Laimbacher J, Vollrath M, Gnehm HE, Sennhauser FH. Brief report: posttraumatic stress disorder in parents of children with newly diagnosed type 1 diabetes. J Pediatric Psychol. 2002;27(7):647–52.

Monaghan M, Horn IB, Alvarez V, Cogen FR, Streisand R. Authoritative parenting, parenting stress, and self-care in pre-adolescents with type 1 diabetes. J Clin Psychol Med Set. 2012;19:255–61.

National Scientific Council on the Developing Child. Young children develop in an environment of relationships. Working Paper No. 1. 2004. http://www.developingchild.net. Accessed 15 Mar 2015.

Padilla-Walker LM, Nelson LJ. Black Hawk Down? Establishing helicopter parenting as a distinct construct from other forms of parental control during emerging adulthood. J Adolesc. 2012;35:1177–90.

Pomerantz EM, Eaton MM. Developmental differences in children's conceptions of parental control: "they love me, but they make me feel incompetent." Merrill Palmer Quart. 2000;46:140–67.

Pomerantz EM, Moorman EA, Litwack SD. The how, whom, and why of parents' involvement in children's academic lives: more is not always better. Rev Educ Res. 2007;77:373–410.

Powers SW, Byars KC, Mitchell MJ, Patton SR, Standiford DA, Dolan LM. Parent report of mealtime behavior and parenting stress in young children with type 1 diabetes and in healthy control subjects. Diabetes C. 2002;25(2):313–8.

Resnick MD, Bearman PS, Blum RW, Bauman KE, Harris KM, Jones J, Joyce T, et al. Protecting adolescents from harm: findings from the National Longitudinal Study on Adolescent Health. JAMA. 1997;278:823–32.

Sabate E. Adherence to long-term therapies: evidence for action. Geneva: World Health Organization; 2003.

Schiffrin H, Liss M, Miles-McLean H, Geary KA, Erchull MJ, Tashner T. Helping or hovering? the effects of helicopter parenting on college students' well-being. J Child Fam Stud. 2013; 23: 548–557.

Schwartz OS, Byrne ML, Simmons JG, Whittle S, Dudgeon P, Sheeber LS, Allen NB. Parenting during early adolescence and adolescent onset major depression: a six-year prospective longitudinal study. Clin Psychol Sci. 2014; 2: 272–286.

Seiffge-Krenke I, Laursen B, Dickson DJ, Hartl AC. Declining metabolic control and decreasing parental support among families with adolescents with diabetes: the risk of restrictiveness. J Pediatric Psychol. 2013;38:518–30.

Shorer M, David R, Schoenberg-Taz M, Levavi-Lavi I, Phillip M, Meyerovitch J. Role of parenting style in achieving metabolic control in adolescents with type 1 diabetes. Diabetes C. 2011;34:1735–7.

Silk JS, Morris AS, Kanaya T, Steinberg L. Psychological control and autonomy granting: opposite ends of a continuum or distinct constructs? J Res Adolescence. 2003;13:113–28.

Steinberg, Laurence; Mounts, Nina S.; Lamborn, Susie D.; Dornbusch, Sanford M. Authoritative parenting and adolescent adjustment across varied ecological niches. J Res Adolesc. 1991;1(1):19–36.

Weissberg-Benchell J, Nansel T, Holmbeck G, et al. Generic and diabetes-specific parent–child behaviors and quality of life among youth with type 1 diabetes. J Pediatr Psychol. 2009;34: 977–88.

Whittle S, Simmons JG, Dennison M, Vijayakumar N, Schwartz O, Yap MB, Sheeber L, Allen NB. Positive parenting predicts the development of adolescent brain structure: a longitudinal study. Dev Cognit Neurosci. 2014;8:7–17.

Wiebe DJ, Berg CA, Korbel C, Palmer DL, Beveridge RM, Upchurch R, et al. Children's appraisals of maternal involvement in coping with diabetes: enhancing our understanding of adherence, metabolic control, and quality of life across adolescence. J Pediatric Psychol. 2005;30:167–78.

Young GS, Mintzer LL, Seacord D, Castañeda M, Mesrkhani V, Stuber ML. Symptoms of posttraumatic stress disorder in parents of transplant recipients: incidence, severity, and related factors. Pediatrics. 2003;111(6):e725–31.

Chapter 8
Poverty, Stress, and Chronic Illness Management

Abstract The burden of illness and the costs of nonadherence fall hardest on impoverished children, who often lack the social, financial, and environmental resources to allow them and their families to manage a chronic illness effectively. Poverty is a societal issue that has plagued humans from the earliest days of civilization, and by many accounts it has gotten worse over the past 10 years in the US. As such, many healthcare providers despair of ever helping their poorest patients struggling with adherence. In this chapter we review the barriers to adherence faced by these vulnerable families, and then discuss their differential exposure to social and environmental stress, which in the worst cases can become "toxic," severely limiting the ability to care for day to day needs. We review the evidence on toxic stress and its implications for chronic illness management. The chapter concludes with a discussion of ways to ameliorate the impact of chronic stress, and the potential of these strategies to improve the adherence and well-being of impoverished children.

According to the World Health Organization (2005), the poor "are most at risk of developing chronic diseases and dying prematurely from them." Poor children have greater exposure to environmental risks and reduced access to health services. They also have poorer adherence to medical regimens, and hence worse illness control (Adler et al. 1994).

Poverty reduces families' abilities to manage the time-consuming complexities and shoulder the effort of managing a chronic illness. Most obviously, poor families have access to fewer resources. They are more likely to lack insurance or be underinsured, reducing their access to primary and preventive care. High out-of-pocket costs (Rector and Venus 2004) and changes or delays in insurance coverage can affect families' ability to fill or refill prescriptions. They have smaller and less beneficial social networks to provide outside support and link them to other resources (Evans 2004). Lower parent education and health literacy can make it more difficult for poor parents to navigate the medical system and follow their children's medical regimens (DeWalt and Hink 2009).

Poor families are also more likely to be single-parent families, and children of single parents are at exceptionally high risk for problematic adherence, even when controlling for socioeconomic factors and minority status (Schwartz et al. 2010; Thompson et al. 2001). Working parents often have very limited options for day-

© Springer International Publishing Switzerland 2015   101
D. D. Schwartz, M. E. Axelrad, *Healthcare Partnerships for Pediatric Adherence*,
SpringerBriefs in Public Health, DOI 10.1007/978-3-319-13668-4_8

care, and many jobs make little or no provision for family leave (National Scientific Council on the Developing Child 2004). As a result, children are often left on their own, unsupervised, for extended periods of time, and for a child with a chronic illness this means having little parent support for illness management—another substantial risk factor for nonadherence, as we discuss in Chaps. 7 and 10.

Resource limitations associated with poverty are generally seen as policy and pragmatic issues rather than clinical concerns. Attempts to address the impact of these problems on adherence have included providing expanded insurance coverage through the Affordable Care Act, enhanced prescription coverage and elimination of out-of-pocket copayments (Choudhry et al. 2011), providing targeted education to high-risk families with low health literacy, calls for improved childcare options for poor families (National Scientific Council on the Developing Child 2004), and the move to umbrella care that includes social and psychological services under the auspices of the medical home. These are certainly beneficial moves with the potential to reduce disparities in healthcare.

However, even if all of the above changes were fully implemented, they would not address one of the fundamental differences between impoverished and higher income families—the substantial exposure to often severe social and environmental stress. As noted by Evans (2004), "Cumulative rather than singular exposure to a confluence of psychosocial and physical environmental risk factors is a potentially critical aspect of the environment of childhood poverty.... exposure to multiple stressors may be a unique, key feature of the environment of childhood poverty" (Evans 2004). Living with chronic stress is likely an important though under-recognized contributor to poverty-linked disparities in pediatric adherence, as discussed in the next section.

Toxic Stress

Child development is an active process that results from an interaction between the child and environmental factors and experiences (De Civita and Dobkin 2004). Most experiences contribute to growth (when the child successfully navigates the experience); however, when an experience is negative and either traumatic or unremitting, and the child has little control over what happens, development can be arrested or affected for the worse.

Stress can be conceived of as any experience that exerts a type of "force" or strain on a person's functioning or development. Current models view stress as either contributing to or impeding development, depending on both the type of stress and on moderating factors. The National Scientific Council on the Developing Child has created a taxonomy of three different stress responses in children that differ in terms of the response's intensity, duration, and ability to disrupt development (including neurodevelopment) (National Scientific Council on the Developing Child 2004).

Positive stress results from stressful experiences to which the child adapts, contributing to growth. Examples include the first day of class, meeting someone new, taking a test, performing in front of others, or managing other challenges. Positive stress is an important ongoing contributor to development and is part of the daily lives of all children. However, some children with significant problems with anxiety avoid sources of positive stress, limiting their developmental progress. Having a chronic illness can sometimes contribute to this avoidance. For example, a diabetic child who has an insulin pump may avoid going to summer camp because of fears of her diabetes being discovered. When anxious children are diagnosed with a new chronic illness, it is important to assess whether they begin to withdraw from participating in developmentally-appropriate growth experiences.

Tolerable stress results from an adverse experience to which the child is still able to adapt. Common examples are the death of a loved one or other loss, an accident, injury, or other frightening experience. New diagnosis of a chronic illness can also result in tolerable stress. The moderating effects of parental support and warm family relationships are critically important to making stress tolerable.

Toxic stress results from adverse childhood experiences (ACEs) that are traumatic or unremitting, and over which the child has little control. Examples include abuse, neglect, exposure to violence, or living with a substance-abusing parent. Poverty is also increasingly seen as source of chronic and possibly toxic stress (Pechtel and Pizzagalli 2010). If the stress is prolonged or severe enough, and parents are unable to buffer the child or provide ways to help the child manage stress, the neurological stress response system (the hypothalamic-pituitary-adrenal axis) gets "set" in such a way as to be more reactive to future stress, and to have more difficulty "shutting off." Children from impoverished backgrounds are exposed to significantly more stress than other children, with fewer resources to help them cope. In consequence, they are more likely to struggle to adapt if they are diagnosed with a chronic illness.

All types of stress result in activation of the autonomic stress response system, causing elevation of heart rate and blood pressure, and production of stress hormones such as cortisol, norepinephrine, and adrenaline (the so-called *fight or flight response*). In response to both positive and tolerable stress, this activation is a temporary condition that returns to baseline once the stressful experience has ended. Not so with toxic stress. Toxic stress results in chronic over-activation of this system, which can result in dysregulation of the stress response itself (precipitating poor responses to stress in the future), and in severe cases can damage the CNS, affecting cognitive, social, and emotional development. Exposure to extreme stress alters the structure and functioning of the amygdala, hippocampus, and prefrontal cortex (McEwen and Gianaros 2011), resulting in increased anxiety and reduced control of mood and memory (Shonkoff et al. 2012).

In fact, there is accruing evidence that toxic stress contributes to a host of serious social ills, including racial/ethnic disparities in cognitive development and educational attainment (Shonkoff 2010), greatly increased incidence in health-risk behaviors (smoking, alcohol, and drug abuse, earlier sexual activity and promiscuous sex), mental health problems such as depression, anxiety (Anda et al. 2006), and risk for suicide (CDC 2006); somatic complaints including obesity and sleep disturbance; high perceived stress, anger problems, and violence (Anda et al. 2006), and medical conditions such as chronic obstructive pulmonary disease, ischemic heart disease, and liver disease (CDC 2006) (Fig. 8.1).

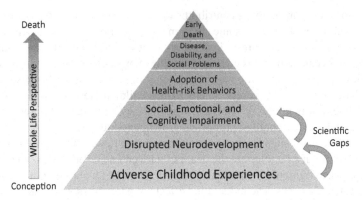

Fig. 8.1 The ACE pyramid. http://www.cdc.gov/violenceprevention/acestudy/pyramid.html

According to CDC (2014; http://www.cdc.gov/violenceprevention/acestudy/prevalence.html), 64% of adults in the original ACE Study sample ($n = 17,337$) reported having experienced one or more ACE in their life, and Garner has suggested that the average pediatrician will see 2–4 children with an ACE score of 4 or higher every day. Thus, this is a problem of astounding magnitude; and there is no doubt that the poor are exposed to higher rates of adverse experiences and toxic stress. According to Child Trend's analysis of data from the 2011/2012 National Survey of Children's Health (2013; http://www.childtrends.org), approximately 12–14% of poor and near-poor children experienced three or more ACEs, compared to only 6% of children at twice the poverty level or higher. As noted above, poor children are also much more likely to develop a chronic illness. For children who have both high toxic stress exposure and a chronic illness, the combination is likely to prove overwhelming (Anderson 2012).

Adaptation to Stress

Even when exposed to severe stressors, most people adapt reasonably well, without experiencing toxic stress or going on to develop more serious outcomes such as post traumatic stress disorder (PTSD). *Diathesis/stress* models posit that certain intrinsic factors (diatheses) predispose someone to greater or lesser vulnerability to stressful situations (Zuckerman 1999). Having a genetic predisposition to depression would be one example. Early exposure to toxic stress is another critically important contributor to stress vulnerability (Anda et al. 2006). As we discussed earlier, chronic illness can be a significant source of stress that can be experienced as traumatic (at diagnosis) and unremitting (as in the case of illnesses like diabetes that require daily management and allow no "holidays").

In many cases even severe stressors can be modulated by parental warmth and support, serving to "detoxify" extreme stress to some degree (National Scientific Council on the Developing Child 2004); but when support is lacking, vulnerability to the affects of stress can be quite high. The role of parents in moderating stress further highlights the importance of parenting to the adjustment (and ultimately adherence behaviors) of children with chronic illness, as will be discussed further below.

Does Toxic Stress Contribute to Nonadherence?

The impact of toxic stress also falls especially heavily on the poor and minorities, contributing to disparities in development, educational and occupational attainment, and both mental and physical health (Shonkoff 2010). We believe that toxic stress is also likely an important contributor to disparities in chronic illness management among impoverished and minority children. Toxic stress could potentially affect adherence in multiple ways.

First, toxic stress can directly affect chronic illness control Stress is associated with increased hyperglycemia in diabetes (Brand et al. 1986; Goetsch 1989), pain episodes in sickle cell disease (Gil et al. 2003; Steinberg 1999), physical malaise in juvenile rheumatic disease (Schanberg et al. 2000), and asthma morbidity (Williams et al. 2009). In the National Cooperative Inner-City Asthma Study ($n = 1528$), 50% of caregivers reported clinically significant symptoms of psychological distress, and on average reported experiencing more than 8 undesirable life events in the preceding 12 months (Wade et al. 1997), and children whose caretakers had clinically significant mental health problems had almost twice as many asthma hospitalizations (Weil et al. 1999). High prevalence of violence in their communities was also associated with asthma morbidity (Wright et al. 2004).

Poor chronic illness control in turn can make adherence much more challenging (Bender and Klinnert 1998; DiMatteo et al. 2007). Patients can end up feeling helpless and hopeless when faced with unresponsive and unremitting symptoms and eventually "give up" on attempts to manage their illness (Polonsky 1996). As suggested by DiMatteo et al. (2007), "Establishing medication and treatment routines central to the management of complex regimens, and attempting to live normal gratifying lives despite the demands of serious disease, can be very difficult when health status becomes increasingly poor."

Second, toxic stress can affect adherence indirectly by reducing a person's ability to engage in self-care or care of a child Toxic stress is strongly (and prospectively) associated with depression, substance abuse (Anda et al. 2006), and risk for suicide (CDC 2006). Depressed individuals often have difficulty with initiative and motivation, and experience fatigue and concentration difficulties, making self-care and chronic illness care much more challenging (Gonzalez et al. 2008), and youth with suicidal ideation have a three-fold increase in nonadherence (Goldston et al. 1997). Alcohol and drug abuse have also been found to be associated with poorer adherence (e.g., Ahmed et al. 2006; Hendershot et al. 2009; Hinkin et al. 2004).

In addition to mental health and behavioral concerns, toxic stress is also associated with cognitive difficulties that can influence adherence. Early in life, toxic stress affects brain development and is believed to be a potent contributor to disparities in learning and cognitive functioning (Baker et al. 2013; Pechtel and Pizzagalli 2010; Shonkoff 2010); including significant memory impairment (Anda et al. 2006) and executive dysfunction (Bos et al. 2009), abilities which are integral to successful illness management (Duke and Harris 2014; Soutor et al. 2004). Memory impairment is especially notable, given that the most common reason offered for medication nonadherence is forgetting (e.g., Buchanan et al. 2012).

Third, toxic stress may affect adherence through an increase in risk-taking behavior Toxic stress is also associated with greatly increased incidence of risk-taking behaviors. As noted above, teens (and adults) with a history of adverse childhood experiences (ACEs) are more likely to abuse alcohol and drugs (Anda et al. 2006). Other risky behaviors associated with early ACEs include smoking, overeating, promiscuous sex (Shonkoff 2010), and gambling (Scherrer et al. 2007). It has been suggested that these behaviors all have the function of reducing stress (which has been termed *behavioral allostasis*; Garner 2013; see also Rothman et al. 2008). However, it is also possible that toxic stress reduces capacity for self-regulation and self control. Indeed, there is evidence that brain areas associated with self-regulation and risk-taking in adolescence are altered in response to toxic stress (McEwen and Gianaros 2011).

The research reviewed above provides a strong albeit circumstantial case for the effect of toxic stress on pediatric adherence. However, there is also some direct evidence that toxic stress can impair adherence. Stressful life events have been found to be associated with lower adherence in children with HIV (Williams et al. 2006), while a history of childhood abuse is a very strong predictor of nonadherence and graft failure in liver transplant patients (Lurie et al. 2000; Shemesh et al. 2007).

Managing Toxic Stress

In a classic article on the effects of poverty on children's psychological functioning, Evans (2004) wrote:

> Psychologists are aware of the multiple disadvantages accompanying low income in America. Yet the search for explanatory processes of poverty's impacts on children has focused almost exclusively on psychosocial characteristics within the family, particularly negative parenting.

He rightly goes on to criticize this focus as too limited, suggesting that it ignores the cumulative exposure to multiple stressors and environmental risk factors that poor children routinely face. While we agree that parenting is not the cause of health disparities—that parenting is not the problem—it is unquestionably a critical part of the solution.

Healthy relationships provide the strongest buffers for childhood adversity (National Scientific Council on the Developing Child 2004). *Positive parenting*—defined as parenting that is supportive and warm—is strongly associated with children's development, behavioral functioning, and psychological well-being

(O. S. Schwartz et al. 2013). As we discuss in Chap. 7, positive parenting is also associated with better regimen adherence, although what constitutes effective parenting changes at different ages.

Comorbid Risk

Finally, it also should be noted that impoverished children and their families are more likely to have multiple risk factors that can interact to further complicated adherence. In one study (Schwartz et al. 2011), children with type 1 diabetes and behavior problems who came from single-parent families (but not those living in dual parent households) had an almost six-fold increase in risk for a diabetes-related emergency room visit post-diagnosis. It may simply be too difficult for single parents to gain compliance from behaviorally difficult children in the face of all of the other competing demands vying for their attention. This finding reinforces two points: that parent-child interactions are a critical determinant of adherence and illness control, and that these interactions (and their outcomes) are strongly influenced by broader macrosystem factors (Bronfenbrenner 1979). To the latter point, in another study examining risk factors in children with type 1 diabetes (Schwartz et al. 2014), patients at moderate risk for developing poor glycemic control had a high incidence of demographic risk factors only, whereas high risk patients had both demographic *and* psychosocial risk (Fig. 8.2.).

Conclusions

Due to the persistence of poverty-related disparities in healthcare utilization, parent education, and health literacy, many clinicians despair of helping their low income patients when problems with adherence emerge. It simply feels like the problems are too big, and too much out of their hands. Poverty is first and foremost a societal

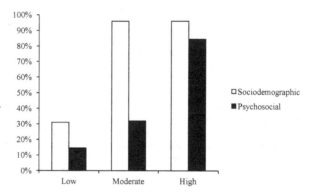

Fig. 8.2 Incidence of risk factors by risk category, collapsed across risk type: sociodemographic risk (Medicaid, single-parent, large family, caregiver unemployed) and psychosocial risk (child behavior, mood, or social problems; family conflict; parent stress/anxiety). (From Schwartz et al. 2014)

and political issue, and progress in addressing poverty-related health disparities in the U.S. has been limited. There are some very promising changes occurring, such as the move to the medical home model, that have the potential to transform healthcare for the poor. Yet the effects of poverty are likely to remain potent for a long time to come.

However, there is a growing recognition that pediatricians and other clinicians do have an important role to play in identifying and managing toxic stress in their patients. The American Academy of Pediatrics has identified toxic stress as a priority area (Garner et al. 2012), and a work group is currently developing guidelines for prevention, screening, and treatment, and for parent education. The AAP recommends public outreach for preventive efforts, in-office screening, and collaborating with networks of other professionals (social workers, psychologists) in treatment. Importantly (we believe critically), the guidelines also stress promotion of the role of positive parenting:

> Because the essence of toxic stress is the absence of buffers needed to return the physiologic stress response to baseline, the primary prevention of its adverse consequences includes those aspects of routine anticipatory guidance that strengthen a family's social supports, encourage a parent's adoption of positive parenting techniques, and facilitate a child's emerging social, emotional, and language skills. (Garner et al. 2012)

As discussed in Chap. 7, interventions focused on positive parenting skills—and collaboration to this end between parents and pediatricians—will likely also prove integral to efforts to improve pediatric adherence.

References

Adler NE, Boyce T, Chesney MA, et al. Socioeconomic status and health. The challenge of the gradient. Am Psychol. 1994;49:15–24.

Ahmed AT, Karter AJ, Liu J. Alcohol consumption is inversely associated with adherence to diabetes self-care behaviours. Diabet Med. 2006;23(7):795–802.

Anda RF, et al. The enduring effects of abuse and related experiences in childhood: a convergence of evidence from neurobiology and epidemiology. Eur Arch Psychiatry Clin Neurosci. 2006;256:174–86.

Anderson BJ. Who forgot? The challenges of family responsibility for adherence in vulnerable pediatric populations. Pediatrics. 2012;129(5):e1324–5.

Baker LM, Williams LM, Korgaonkar MS, Cohen RA, Heaps JM, Paul RH. Impact of early versus late childhood early stress on brain morphometrics. Brain Imag Behav. 2013;7:196–203.

Bender BG, Klinnert MD. Psychological correlates of asthma severity and treatment outcome in children. In: Kotses H, Harver A, editors. Self-management of asthma. New York: Marcel Dekker; 1998. pp. 63–88.

Bos KJ, Fox N, Zeanah CH, Nelson CA. Effects of early psychosocial deprivation on the development of memory and executive function. Front Behav Neurosci. 2009;3(16):1–7.

Brand AH, Johnson JH, Johnson SB. Life stress and indicators of diabetic control in children with insulin-dependent diabetes. J Pediatr Psychol. 1986;11:481–95.

Bronfenbrenner U. The ecology of human development: experiments by nature and design. Cambridge: Harvard University Press; 1979.

Buchanan AL, Montepiedra G, Sirois PA, et al. Barriers to medication adherence in HIV-infected children and youth based on self- and caregiver report. Pediatrics. 2012;129(5):e1244–e1251.

Centers for Disease Control and Prevention. Atlanta: CDC; 2006. Adverse Childhood Experiences Study. http://www.cdc.gov/nccdphp/ace/index.htm. Accessed 16 Mar 2015.

Centers for Disease Control and Prevention. http://www.cdc.gov/violenceprevention/acestudy/findings.html. last updated May 2014. Accessed 16 Mar 2015.

Choudhry NK, et al. Full coverage for preventive medications after myocardial infarction. N Engl J Med. 2011;365:2088–97.

De Civita M, Dobkin PL. Pediatric adherence as a multidimensional and dynamic construct, involving a triadic partnership. J Pediatr Psychol. 2004;29:157–69.

DeWalt DA, Hink A. Health literacy and child health outcomes: a systematic review of the literature. Pediatrics. 2009;124:S265–74.

DiMatteo MR, Haskard KB, Williams SL. Health beliefs, disease severity, and patient adherence: a meta-analysis. Med Care. 2007;45:521–8.

Duke DC, Harris MA. Executive function, adherence, and glycemic control in adolescents with type 1 diabetes: a literature review. Curr Diab Rep. 2014;14(10):532.

Evans GW. The environment of childhood poverty. Am Psychol. 2004;59(2):77–92.

Garner AS, et al. Early childhood adversity, toxic stress, and the role of the pediatrician: translating developmental science into lifelong health. Pediatrics. 2012;129:e224–31.

Gil KM, Carson JW, Porter LS, Ready J, Valrie C, Redding-Lallinger R, Daeschner C. Daily stress and mood and their association with pain, health-care use, and school activity in adolescents with sickle cell disease. J Pediatr Psychol. 2003;28(5):363–73.

Goetsch VL. Stress and blood glucose in diabetes mellitus: a review and methodological commentary. Ann Behav Med. 1989;11(3):102–7.

Goldston DB, Kelley AE, Reboussin DM, et al. Suicidal ideation and behaviour and noncompliance with the medical regimen among diabetic adolescents. J Am Acad Child Adol Psychiat. 1997;36:1528–36.

Gonzalez JS, Peyrot M, McCarl LA, et al. Depression and diabetes treatment non-adherence: a meta-analysis. Diabetes Care. 2008;31:2398–403.

Hendershot CS, Stoner SA, Pantalone DW, Simoni JM. Alcohol use and antiretroviral adherence: review and meta-analysis. J Acquir Immune Defic Syndr (1999). 2009;52(2):180.

Hinkin CH, Hardy DJ, Mason KI, Castellon SA, Durvasula RS, Lam MN, Stefaniak M. Medication adherence in HIV-infected adults: effect of patient age, cognitive status, and substance abuse. AIDS (Lond, Engl). 2004;18(Suppl 1):S19.

Lurie S, Shemesh E, Sheiner PA, Emre S, Tindle HL, Melchionna L, Schneider BL. Non-adherence in pediatric liver transplant recipients—an assessment of risk factors and natural history. Pediatr Transplant. 2000;4(3):200–6.

McEwen BS, Gianaros PJ. Stress- and allostasis-induced brain plasticity. Annu Rev Med. 2011;62:431–45.

National Scientific Council on the Developing Child 2004. Young children develop in an environment of relationships. Working Paper No. 1. http://www.developingchild.net (2004). Accessed 16 Mar 2015.

National Scientific Council on the Developing Child. Excessive stress disrupts the architecture of the developing brain: working paper #3. developing-child.harvard.edu/resources/reports_and_working_papers/. Accessed 16 Mar 2015.

National Survey of Children's Health (July 2013). http://www.childtrends.org/?indicators=adverse-experiences. Accessed 16 Mar 2015.

Pechtel P, Pizzagalli D. Effects of early life stress on cognitive and affective function: an integrated review of human literature. Psychopharmacology. 2010;214:1–3.

Polonsky WH. Understanding and treating patients with diabetes burnout. Practical psychology for diabetes clinicians. Alexandria: American Diabetes Association; 1996. pp. 183–92.

Rector TS, Venus PJ. Do drug benefits help Medicare beneficiaries afford prescribed drugs? Health Aff (Millwood). 2004;23:213–22.

Rothman EF, Edwards EM, Heeren T, Hingson RW. Adverse childhood experiences predict earlier age of drinking onset: results from a representative US sample of current or former drinkers. Pediatrics. 2008;122(2):e298–e304.

Schanberg LE, Sandstrom MJ, Starr K, Gil KM, Lefebvre JC, Keefe FJ, et al. The relationship of daily mood and stressful events to symptoms in juvenile rheumatic disease. Arthritis Care Res. 2000;13:33.

Scherrer JF, Xian H, Kapp JM, et al. Association between exposure to childhood and lifetime traumatic events and lifetime pathological gambling in a twin cohort. J Nerv Ment Dis. 2007;195(1):72–78pmid:17220743.

Schwartz DD, Cline VD, Hansen J, Axelrad ME, Anderson BJ. Early risk factors for nonadherence in pediatric type 1 diabetes: a review of the recent literature. Curr Diabetes Rev. 2010;6:167–83.

Schwartz DD, Cline VD, Axelrad ME, Anderson BJ. Feasibility, acceptability, and predictive validity of a psychosocial screening program for children and youth newly diagnosed with Type 1 diabetes. Diabetes Care. 2011;34:326–31.

Schwartz OS, Byrne ML, Simmons JG, Whittle S, Dudgeon P, Sheeber LS, Allen NB. Parenting during early adolescence and adolescent onset major depression: a six-year prospective longitudinal study. Clin Psychol Sci. 2013.

Schwartz, DD, Axelrad ME, Anderson BJ. A psychosocial risk index for poor glycemic control in children and adolescents with Type 1 diabetes. Pediatr Diabetes 2014; 15: 190–197.

Shemesh E, Annunziato RA, Yehuda R, Schneider BL, Newcorn JH, Hutson C, Cohen JA, Briere J, Gorman JM, Emre S. Childhood abuse, nonadherence, and medical outcome in pediatric liver transplant recipients. J Am Acad Child Adolesc Psychiat. 2007;46(10):1280–9.

Shonkoff JP. Building a new bio- developmental framework to guide the fu- ture of early childhood policy. Child Dev. 2010;81:357–67.

Shonkoff JP, Garner AS, Siegel BS, Dobbins MI, Earls MF, McGuinn L, Pascoe J, Wood DL. The lifelong effects of early childhood adversity and toxic stress. Pediatrics. 2012;129:e232–46.

Soutor SA, Chen R, Streisand R, Kaplowitz P, Holmes CS. Memory matters: developmental differences in predictors of diabetes care behaviors. J Pediatr Psychol. 2004;29:493–505.

Steinberg MH. Management of sickle cell disease. N Engl J Med. 1999;340(13):1021–30.

Thompson SJ, Auslander WF, White NH. Comparison of single-mother and two-parent families on metabolic control of children with diabetes. Diabetes Care. 2001;24:234–8.

Wade S, Weil C, Holden G, et al. Psychosocial characteristics of inner-city children with asthma: a description of the NCICAS psychosocial protocol. Pediatr Pulmonol. 1997;24(4):263–76.

Weil CM, et al. The relationship between psychosocial factors and asthma morbidity in Inner-City children with asthma. Pediatrics. 1999;104(6):1274–80.

Williams PL, Storm D, Montepiedra G, Nichols S, Kammer B, Sirois PA, et al. Predictors of adherence to antiretroviral medications in children and adolescents with HIV infection. Pediatrics. 2006;118:e1745–57.

Williams DR, Sternthal M, Wright RJ. Social determinants: taking the social context of asthma seriously. Pediatrics. 2009;123;S174.

World Health Organization 2005. Preventing Chronic Diseases: A Vital Investment. World Health Organization. http://www.who.int/chp/chronic_disease_report/en/. Accessed 16 Mar 2015.

Wright RJ, Mitchell H, Visness CM, Cohen S, Stout J, Evans R, Gold DR. Community violence and asthma morbidity: the Inner-City asthma study. Am J Public Health. 2004;94(4):625–32.

Zuckerman M. Vulnerability to psychopathology: a biosocial model. Washington, DC: American Psychological Association; 1999.

Chapter 9
Racial/Ethnic Disparities and Adherence

Ashley Butler

Abstract This chapter describes the pervasiveness of racial/ethnic disparities in outcomes of pediatric chronic conditions, and focuses on low adherence to treatment regimens among minority children and their families as a contributor to these disparities. We emphasize the need to increase effective parent- and adolescent-provider communication within a health system approach to promote adherence among minority children. We discuss ways that providers, parents, and adolescents can build skills to achieve effective communication. Finally, we describe the importance of a culturally competent workforce to help minority parents and adolescents build effective skills for communicating with providers to promote adherence.

Overview of Health Disparities among Racial/Ethnic Minority Children

The term *health disparity population* is defined by the National Institute on Minority Health and Health Disparities (NIMHD) as a group that experiences a significant disparity in the overall rate of disease incidence, prevalence, morbidity, mortality, or survival rates compared to the health status of the general population. Racial/ethnic minorities in the U.S. are designated as one health disparity population and consist of the following groups: African Americans, American Indians/Alaska Natives, Asians, Hispanics, and Native Hawaiians and Other Pacific Islanders.

While most research and national attention has focused on health disparities among minority adults, disparities in children's health are also extensive, pervasive and persistent (Flores and the Committee on Pediatric Research 2010). Research has detailed disparities in overall mortality rates, prevention, and general health status of children, (Flores and the Committee on Pediatric Research 2010) and these differences generally persist when other, correlated factors such as SES are controlled. Moreover, minorities, especially African Americans, have greater exposure

A. Butler (✉)
Department of Pediatrics, Section of Psychology,
Baylor College of Medicine, Houston, Texas, USA
e-mail: ambutler@texaschildrens.org

© Springer International Publishing Switzerland 2015
D. D. Schwartz, M. E. Axelrad, *Healthcare Partnerships for Pediatric Adherence,*
SpringerBriefs in Public Health, DOI 10.1007/978-3-319-13668-4_9

to toxic stress (http://www.childtrends.org/wp-content/uploads/2013/07/124_Adverse_Experiences.pdf) which can have a substantial impact on medical adherence.

Studies have also concentrated on the outcomes of chronic conditions among minority children. Unfortunately, minority children disproportionately experience adverse outcomes in a number of chronic conditions (Berry et al. 2010). African American and Puerto Rican children have higher asthma mortality rates compared to non-Hispanic white children. Diabetes-related death among African American children is twice the rate of non-Hispanic white youth (CDC 2007). There are shorter survival rates for some congenital heart conditions among African American children (Boneva et al. 2001) and for Acute Leukemia among Hispanic children (Linabery and Ross 2008). American Indian and African American children with attention-deficit hyperactivity disorder (ADHD) have 4 times higher odds of school failure and 11 times higher odds of family burden compared to non-minority children (Ezpeleta et al. 2001). Compared to the many studies that have described disparities in children's health outcomes, a much smaller body of literature has focused on modifiable factors that influence child health disparities or solutions to eliminate them.

Racial/ethnic differences in various characteristics of health care are included in most models to explain disparities in health outcomes and to guide the development of strategies for disparities reduction (Kilbourne et al. 2006). Differences in the health care outcomes across racial/ethnic groups are likely due to the interaction of patient (and parent)-, provider-, and health system factors. The higher rate of nonadherence to treatment regimens among minority children is one consequence of inequity in health care that contributes to disparities in health outcomes among minority children with chronic conditions.

Adherence among Racial/Ethnic Minority Children

Poorer adherence to treatment recommendations among minority children compared to non-minority children has been documented for a number of chronic conditions. African American and Hispanic children with asthma are less likely to adhere to clinic visits or use inhaled corticosteroids (Crocker et al. 2009). These groups of children also are less likely to use medication for ADHD (Saloner et al. 2013) and for depression (Fontanella et al. 2011). Children with type 1 diabetes have significantly poorer glycemic control (Mayer-Davis et al. 2009; Schwartz et al. 2013) that is at least partly attributable to lower overall adherence to the diabetes regimen (Auslander et al. 1997). Auslander et al. reported less frequent blood glucose checking and poorer dietary adherence among diabetic African American youth. Schwartz et al. (Schwartz et al. 2011) found that African American families were significantly more likely to miss diabetes clinic follow-up appointments than other groups. Over 65% missed one or more appointments in the first nine months following diagnosis, compared to 41% of Hispanic families and 24% of Caucasian families. Hispanic children have demonstrated lower adherence to oral mediation for type 2 diabetes (Adeyemi et al. 2012) and to medication treatment for Acute

Lymphoblastic Leukemia compared to non-minority children (Bhatia et al. 2012). African American children showed higher nonadherence to antiretroviral treatment for human immunodeficiency virus (Naar-King et al. 2013) and to medication for hypertension (Eakin et al. 2013).

Given the widespread disparities in nonadherence, we emphasize that improving adherence among minority children is an essential goal to help eliminate disparities in outcomes of chronic conditions. Below we describe the potential of enhancing parent-, adolescent-, and provider communication for improving adherence among minority children.

Parent- and Adolescent-Provider Communication and Adherence

Many studies show that effective patient-provider communication is associated with higher adherence to treatment regimens (Zolnierek and Dimatteo 2009). For example, when providers elicit parent participation in asthma treatment plans, children are more adherent to asthma medication 1 month later (Sleath et al. 2012). Experts have indicated that ineffective communication between minority parents, minority adolescents, and their providers also contributes to racial and ethnic differences in adherence. Health communication theory provides a conceptual model for explaining the role of communication in racial/ethnic differences in treatment adherence.

Ashton and colleagues (Ashton et al. 2003) set forth a health communication conceptual framework that is grounded in the *explanatory model of illness* (Kleinman et al. 1978). The explanatory model of illness postulates that patients and providers each have their own unique perceptions of health conditions and treatment options. Explanatory models of illness can greatly vary between providers and patients from different racial/ethnic and cultural groups. Ashton et al. argue that effective communication is especially needed to develop a *shared explanatory model of health* conditions between patients and providers from different groups, and thereby to promote treatment adherence (Ashton et al. 2003).

Empirical studies support this model by demonstrating racial/ethnic differences in effective parent- and adolescent- provider communication. Parents of minority children with chronic physical conditions report less participation in treatment decision making than non-minority parents (Butler et al. 2014). Providers give less information about medication options, are more likely to use impersonal biomedical language (Roter et al. 1997) and less likely to elicit preferences, expectations, or concerns among African American parents compared to non-minority parents (Brinkman et al. 2011). Providers also direct fewer questions to African American and Hispanic youth compared to non-minority youth (Stivers and Majid 2007). Several cultural, perceptual, and educational factors likely influence less effective communication patterns between providers and minority parents and adolescents.

Factors that Influence Communication Between Minority Families and Healthcare Providers

Ashton et al. posit that differences in language (terms, idioms, and metaphors to describe health), styles of communicating, or perceptions of balance, power, and trust in the patient-provider interaction may limit the development of a shared model when patients and providers are from different racial/ethnic backgrounds (Ashton et al. 2003). Other researchers have focused on the role of *implicit attitudes* among providers and racial differences in patient-provider communication. Implicit attitudes are those that are outside of awareness, and are not available to report, and are therefore considered "unconscious."

Cooper et al. (2012) examined the relation between primary care clinicians' implicit attitudes about race and their communication with patients and patient ratings of care. Specifically, they used the computer-based Implicit Association Test (IAT; Greenwald et al. 1998) to examine the relative association strength between the target concepts *race* (White vs. Black) and patient *compliance* (e.g., willing, reliable, and helpful vs. reluctant, apathetic, and lax). They hypothesized that negative implicit stereotypes of Black patients as measured by the IAT would be associated with clinicians' nonverbal communication and patient ratings of care. Findings indicated that implicit racial stereotyping was associated with less rapport-building and facilitative communication to obtain the perspective of African American patients, and less rapport-building and facilitative communication was related to lower patient satisfaction with care. At the same time, implicit racial stereotyping among providers was associated with more rapport building and facilitative communication with non-Hispanic white patients, and more rapport building and facilitative communication was associated with greater patient satisfaction with care (Cooper et al. 2012). Cooper et.al concluded that implicit attitudes about race among providers may contribute to ineffective communication among minority patients. Thus, implicit racial attitudes may limit the development of a shared model of health during healthcare interactions with minority families by contributing to less effective communication.

In general, patients and families who perceive discrimination or distrust their provider are more likely not to follow treatment recommendations and tend to have worse health outcomes (Hausmann et al. 2008; Trivedi and Ayanian 2006; Williams 2003). Some research indicates that distrust is more likely when patient and provider are from different racial/ethnic backgrounds (Street et al. 2008), although much of the effect of congruence may be due to communication differences, as noted above (Ashton et al. 2003).

The level of parent and adolescent health literacy or culturally-related health beliefs may also contribute to ineffective communication (Diette and Rand 2007). As noted earlier, *health literacy* is defined as the capacity to obtain, process, and understand basic health information and services needed to make appropriate health decisions (Institute of Medicine 2004). African American and Hispanic parents are more likely to have low health literacy than non-Hispanic white parents (Yin et al. 2009). Lower health literacy among minority parents may be due to lower educational attainment or limited English proficiency.

Finally, a number of studies have shown racial/ethnic differences in health beliefs and perceptions. For example, there are racial/ethnic differences in parental and adolescent beliefs about the causes of child mental health conditions and treatment options (Bussing et al. 2012; Dosreis et al. 2003; Yeh et al. 2004). African American and Hispanic parents of children with asthma have lower expectations for child functioning, stronger perceptions of competing family priorities, and more medication concerns than non-Hispanic white parents (Conn et al. 2007; Wu et al. 2008). Low health literacy or culturally-related health beliefs among minority parents and adolescents may limit effective communication to develop a shared model of health and partnerships with providers. Below we discuss strategies to promote effective communication between minority families and providers.

Promoting Effective Parent-Provider and Adolescent-Provider Communication

To date, most interventions targeting effective patient-provider communication to promote adherence have focused on adult health disparities. We draw on techniques from the adult literature to provide the following recommendations for promoting effective parent-provider communication as a strategy to prevent nonadherence in pediatrics. Research in adult care supports the need to build the skills of parents and adolescents, as well as providers when seeking to enhance effective communication (Alegria et al. 2014).

Communication Skills Training for Providers Communication skills training for providers is recommended to enhance parent-and adolescent-provider communication to promote adherence among minority children. Social cognitive theory suggests that enhancing providers' communication skills that build partnerships with families can prevent or eliminate the impact of implicit attitudes on racial/ethnic differences in communication during health care visits (Burgess et al. 2007). Communication skills training should aim to enhance skills for patient-centered communication and collaborative decision-making to reach the goal of establishing a shared model of health and strong partnerships between providers and minority families.

Parent- and adolescent-centered communication are defined as verbal behaviors that increase providers' understanding of parents' and adolescents' individual needs, perspectives, and values; give them the information they need to participate in their care; and build trust and understanding (Levinson et al. 2010). Parent- and adolescent-centered communication skills include information giving, question asking, supportiveness, and partnership building (Wissow et al. 2011; Horn et al. 2012). *Collaborative decision-making* is the degree to which parents and providers share power when making decisions (Charles et al. 1997).

Table 9.1 provides an example of communication skills training activities and content for providers. Components of in-person communication skills training for

Table 9.1 Communication skills training for providers

Delivery Methods
Didactic presentations/CMEs
Small-group discussion
Guided role play
Written materials
Coaching Activities
Observe demonstration of communication skills
Practice communication skills with simulated parent and adolescent and receive feedback
Complete self-assessment exercises
Review written information on treatment guidelines for health condition (if applicable)
Review written summaries of research on culturally-specific health beliefs and perceived barriers to adherence among minority parents and adolescents
Communication Training Targets
Asking open-ended questions to
Elicit parent and adolescent concerns about the health condition and its treatment
Understand parent and adolescent knowledge and beliefs about the health condition; monitor adherence
Understand parent and adolescent perceptions of barriers to adherence
Providing information about the health condition and treatment in short, clear statements (followed up with brief written materials)
Being supportive by making emotional connections and supportive statements
Building a partnership by engaging both the parent and the adolescent in problem-solving and shared treatment decision-making

providers include didactic instruction, role-play, and individualized feedback to providers based on their interaction with a simulated parent or adolescent. Communication skills training to improve the care of minority patients should also include didactic content and individualized feedback based on simulated interactions that focus on culturally specific health beliefs (e.g., medication concerns, and expectations). Training can occur within small groups, and ideally would include some role-play to practice skills.

Training may also need to concentrate on helping providers assess the health literacy of parents and adolescents, and strategies to tailor health information to their literacy level. For example, successful strategies may include adding video to verbal narratives to deliver important health information. Emerging studies suggest that web-based communication skills training may be a cost-effective and scalable alternative to in-person communication skills training for providers. Specifically, meta-analysis of research in provider medical education suggests that web-based interventions are equivalent to traditional in-person methods for improving knowledge and skill acquisition (Cook et al. 2008).

Coaching for Parents and Adolescents Coaching interventions for adolescents and parents are also encouraged to increase effective communication with pro-

Table 9.2 Communication skills training for patients and parents

Delivery Methods
In clinic
20 min face-to-face pre-encounter coaching session
10 min face-to-face post-encounter debriefing session
Follow-Up
20–30 min phone follow-up session prior to the child's next scheduled appointment
Written materials
Coaching Activities
Discussion of any parent concerns regarding previous interaction with provider and changes they would like to make
Discussion of parent and adolescent concerns and perceived barriers to the management of the chronic condition
Parents and adolescents write down appointment information, treatment regimen, and questions they will ask provider
Parents and adolescents practice disclosing concerns, asking questions, and stating preferences with communication coach
Coach provides reinforcement and reminders about preparing for upcoming visits
Discussion of ways parents and adolescents can obtain support for preparing for upcoming visits with their provider
Parents and adolescents review written stories with graphics (e.g., photo-novels) that depict parent and adolescents using communication skills
Communication Training Targets
Disclosing concerns about health condition and barriers to engaging in treatment regimen
Asking questions to obtain information about health condition and treatment
Stating treatment preferences

viders to prevent nonadherence. Table 9.2 provides an overview of activities that can be completed during coaching sessions with parents and adolescents and the communication skills that can be the focus of sessions. Coaching interventions for parents provide information about the chronic health condition, encourage parental empowerment and active involvement in care, and teach specific strategies for communicating with providers. Coaching sessions teach parents and adolescents effective communication techniques to promote collaborative communication and shared decision making with providers using modeling and role play.

Given the roles of health literacy and culturally related health beliefs (e.g., perceptions of competing demands, medication concerns) in parent-provider communication among minority families, it is important that coaching interventions also address these elements. For example, information about chronic health conditions during coaching sessions may be tailored to the health literacy level of parents and adolescents. Culturally related health beliefs or perceptions can be elicited during coaching sessions, and parents and adolescents can be encouraged to discuss these beliefs with their providers.

Researchers focused on coaching interventions with minority adults have noted the need to ensure coaching interventions are delivered by culturally-competent staff to enhance the credibility, relevance, cultural appropriateness, and effectiveness of such interventions among minority patients (Cooper et al. 2013). One way to do this is through the use of *lay health workers*, individuals who do not have formal healthcare training but receive on the job training. Interventions delivered by lay health workers to families of children with chronic conditions have shown improvements in urgent care use and family psychosocial functioning (Raphael et al. 2013), and there is evidence that coaching sessions delivered by lay health workers may enhance the cultural appropriateness of coaching for minority parents and adolescents. Encouragingly, coaching interventions to enhance partnerships between families and providers as a strategy to promote adherence align with opportunities available through the Patient Protection and Affordable Care Act, which promotes the development of healthcare teams that include lay health workers.

Summary and Conclusions

Racial/ethnic minority children experience disparities in outcomes of chronic conditions that are costly to the health care system and place a significant burden on families. Higher rates of nonadherence to treatment regimens among minority children across a range of chronic conditions contribute to these disparities. Enhancing parent- and adolescent-centered communication and collaborative decision-making between minority families and providers has been shown to increase adherence in adult care among minority adults. Improving communication and collaborative decision making also holds promise for preventing nonadherence in pediatrics.

Recommendations for improving communication among vulnerable families include communication skills training for providers, and coaching interventions for parents and adolescents. Such strategies should emphasize tailoring communication to the health literacy level of vulnerable families, and addressing culturally-related health beliefs. Opportunities available through the Patient Protection and Affordable care Act that focus on wellness and care delivered by lay health workers can serve as a catalyst for strategies to improve healthcare providers' communication with vulnerable minority families.

References

Adeyemi AO, Rascati KL, Lawson KA, Strassels SA. Adherence to oral antidiabetic medications in the pediatric population with type 2 diabetes: a retrospective database analysis. Clin Ther. 2012;34(3):712–9.

Alegria M, Carson N, Flores M, Li X, Shi P, Lessios AS, et al. Activation, self-management, engagement, and retention in behavioral health care: a randomized clinical trial of the DECIDE intervention. JAMA Psychiatry. 2014;7:557–65.

Ashton CM, Haidet P, Paterniti DA, Collins TC, Gordon HS, O'Malley K, et al. Racial and ethnic disparities in the use of health services: bias, preferences, or poor communication? J Gen Intern Med. 2003;18(2):146–5.

Auslander WF, Thompson S, Dreitzer D, White NH, Santiago JV. Disparity in glycemic control and adherence between African-American and Caucasian youths with diabetes: family and community contexts. Diabetes Care. 1997;20:1569–75.

Berry JG, Bloom S, Foley S, Palfrey JS. Health inequity in children and youth with chronic health conditions. Pediatrics. 2010;126(Suppl 3):S111–9.

Bhatia S, Landier W, Shangguan M, Hageman L, Schaible AN, Carter AR, et al. Nonadherence to oral mercaptopurine and risk of relapse in Hispanic and non-Hispanic white children with acute lymphoblastic leukemia: a report from the children's oncology group. J Clin Oncol. 2012;30(17):2094–101.

Boneva RS, Botto LD, Moore CA, Yang Q, Correa A, Erickson JD. Mortality associated with congenital heart defects in the United States: trends and racial disparities, 1979–1997. Circulation. 2001;103(19):2376–81.

Brinkman WB, Hartl J, Rawe LM, Sucharew H, Britto MT, Epstein JN. Physicians' shared decision-making behaviors in attention-deficit/hyperactivity disorder care. Arch Pediatr Adolesc Med. 2011;165(11):1013–9.

Burgess D, van Ryn M, Dovidio J, Saha S. Reducing racial bias among health care providers: lessons from social-cognitive psychology. J Gen Intern Med. 2007;22(6):882–7.

Bussing R, Zima BT, Mason DM, Meyer JM, White K, Garvan CW. ADHD knowledge, perceptions, and information sources: perspectives from a community sample of adolescents and their parents. J Adolesc Health. 2012;51(6):593–600.

Butler AM, Elkins S, Kowalkowski M, Raphael JL. Shared decision making among parents of children with mental health conditions compared to children with chronic physical conditions. Matern Child Health J. 2014;19(2):410–418.

Centers for Disease Control and Prevention. Racial disparities in diabetes mortality among persons aged 1–19 years–United States, 1979–2004. MMWR Morb Mortal Wkly Rep. 2007;56(45):1184–7.

Charles C, Gafni A, Whelan T. Shared decision-making in the medical encounter: what does it mean? (or it takes at least two to tango). Soc Sci Med. 1997;44(5):681–92.

Conn KM, Halterman JS, Lynch K, Cabana MD. The impact of parents' medication beliefs on asthma management. Pediatrics. 2007;120(3):e521–6.

Cook DA, Levinson AJ, Garside S, Dupras DM, Erwin PJ, Montori VM. Internet-based learning in the health professions: a meta-analysis. JAMA. 2008;300(10):1181–96.

Cooper LA, Roter DL, Carson KA, Beach MC, Sabin JA, Greenwald AG, et al. The associations of clinicians' implicit attitudes about race with medical visit communication and patient ratings of interpersonal care. Am J Public Health. 2012;102(5):979–87.

Cooper LA, Ghods Dinoso BK, Ford DE, Roter DL, Primm AB, Larson SM, et al. Comparative effectiveness of standard versus patient-centered collaborative care interventions for depression among African Americans in primary care settings: the BRIDGE Study. Health Serv Res. 2013;48(1):150–74.

Crocker D, Brown C, Moolenaar R, Moorman J, Bailey C, Mannino D, et al. Racial and ethnic disparities in asthma medication usage and health-care utilization: data from the National Asthma Survey. Chest. 2009;136(4):1063–71.

Diette GB, Rand C. The contributing role of health-care communication to health disparities for minority patients with asthma. Chest. 2007;132(5 Suppl):802S–9S.

Dosreis S, Zito JM, Safer DJ, Soeken KL, Mitchell JW Jr, Ellwood LC. Parental perceptions and satisfaction with stimulant medication for attention-deficit hyperactivity disorder. J Dev Behav Pediatr. 2003;24(3):155–62.

Eakin MN, Brady T, Kandasamy V, Fivush B, Riekert KA. Disparities in antihypertensive medication adherence in adolescents. Pediatr Nephrol. 2013;28(8):1267–73.

Ezpeleta L, Keeler G, Erkanli A, Costello EJ, Angold A. Epidemiology of psychiatric disability in childhood and adolescence. J Child Psychol Psychiatry. 2001;42(7):901–14.

Flores G and the Committee on Pediatric Research. Technical report—racial and ethnic disparities in the health and health care of children. Pediatrics. 2010;125:e979–1020.

Fontanella CA, Bridge JA, Marcus SC, Campo JV. Factors associated with antidepressant adherence for medicaid-enrolled children and adolescents. Ann Pharmacother. 2011;45(7–8):898–909.

Greenwald AG, McGhee DE, Schwartz JL. Measuring individual differences in implicit cognition: the implicit association test. J Pers Soc Psychol. 1998;74(6):1464–80.

Hausmann LRM, Kwonho J, Bost JE, Ibrahim SA. Perceived discrimination in health care and health status in a racially diverse sample. Med Care. 2008;46:905–14.

Horn IB, Mitchell SJ, Wang J, Joseph JG, Wissow LS. African-American parents' trust in their child's primary care provider. Acad Pediatr. 2012;12(5):399–404.

Institute of Medicine. Health literacy: a prescription to end confusion. Washington, DC: National Academies Press; 2004.

Kilbourne AM, Switzer G, Hyman K, Crowley-Matoka M, Fine MJ. Advancing health disparities research within the health care system: a conceptual framework. Am J Public Health. 2006;96(12):2113–21.

Kleinman AM, Eisenberg L, Good B. Culture, illness, and care. Clinical lessons from anthropological and cross-cultural research. Ann Intern Med. 1978;88:251–8.

Levinson W, Lesser CS, Epstein RM. Developing physician communication skills for patient-centered care. Health Aff (Millwood) 2010;29(7):1310–8.

Linabery AM, Ross JA. Childhood and adolescent cancer survival in the US by race and ethnicity for the diagnostic period 1975–1999. Cancer. 2008;113(9):2575–96.

Mayer-Davis EJ, Beyer J, Bell RA, Dabelea D, D'Agostino R, Imperatore G, Lawrence JM, et al. Diabetes in African American youth: prevalence, incidence, and clinical characteristics: the SEARCH for diabetes in youth study. Diabetes Care. 2009;32(Suppl 2):S112–22.

Naar-King S, Montepiedra G, Garvie P, Kammerer B, Malee K, Sirois PA, et al. Social ecological predictors of longitudinal HIV treatment adherence in youth with perinatally acquired HIV. J Pediatr Psychol. 2013;38(6):664–74.

Raphael JL, Rueda A, Lion KC, Giordano TP. The role of lay health workers in pediatric chronic disease: a systematic review. Acad Pediatr. 2013;13(5):408–20.

Roter DL, Stewart M, Putnam SM, Lipkin M, Stiles W, Inui TS. Communication styles of primary care physicians. JAMA. 1997;277:350–6.

Saloner B, Fullerton C, McGuire T. The impact of long-acting medications on attention-deficit/hyperactivity disorder treatment disparities. J Child Adolesc Psychopharmacol. 2013;23(6):401–9.

Schwartz DD, Cline VD, Axelrad ME, Anderson BJ. Feasibility, acceptability, and predictive validity of a psychosocial screening program for children and youth newly diagnosed with Type 1 diabetes. Diabetes Care. 2011;34:326–31.

Schwartz DD, Axelrad ME, Anderson BJ. A psychosocial risk index for poor glycemic control in children and adolescents with Type 1 diabetes. Pediatr Diabetes. 2014;15:190–197.

Sleath B, Carpenter DM, Slota C, Williams D, Tudor G, Yeatts K, et al. Communication during pediatric asthma visits and self-reported asthma medication adherence. Pediatrics. 2012;130(4):627–33.

Stivers T, Majid A. Questioning children: interactional evidence of implicit bias in medical interviews. Soc Psychol Q. 2007;70(4):424–41.

Street RL, O'Malley KJ, Cooper LA, Haidet P. Understanding concordance in patient-physician relationships: personal and ethnic dimensions of shared identity. Ann Fam Med. 2008;6:198–205.

Trivedi AN, Ayanian JZ. Perceived discrimination and use of preventive health services. J Gen Intern Med. 2006;21:553–8.

Williams DR, Neighbors HW, Jackson JS. Racial/ethnic discrimination and health: findings from community studies. Am J Public Health. 2003;93:200–8.

Wissow, Gadomski A, Roter D, Larson S, Lewis B, Brown J. Aspects of mental health communication skills training that predict parent and child outcomes in pediatric primary care. Patient Educ Couns. 2011;82(2):226–32.

Wu AC, Smith L, Bokhour B, Hohman KH, Lieu TA. Racial/Ethnic variation in parent perceptions of asthma. Ambul Pediatr. 2008;8(2):89–97.

Yeh M, Hough RL, McCabe K, Lau A, Garland A. Parental beliefs about the causes of child problems: exploring racial/ethnic patterns. J Am Acad Child Adolesc Psychiatry. 2004;43(5):605–12.

Yin HS, Johnson M, Mendelsohn AL, Abrams MA, Sanders LM, Dreyer BP. The health literacy of parents in the United States: a nationally representative study. Pediatrics. 2009;124(Suppl 3):S289–98.

Zolnierek KB, Dimatteo MR. Physician communication and patient adherence to treatment: a meta-analysis. Med Care. 2009;47(8):826–34.

Part II
Implications for Policy and Practice

Chapter 10
Rethinking Self-Management

Abstract Current definitions and conceptualizations of adherence continue to place the primary responsibility for illness management on the patient from the time of adolescence forward, even while acknowledging that successful adherence reflects collaboration between multiple actors. In this chapter we review the push for independent illness management that often accompanies the onset of adolescence, and the evidence for and against independent self-care. We conclude with suggestions for a different approach that focuses on autonomy rather than independence as the most appropriate goal for adolescent illness management.

Much of the literature reviewed so far leads to the same conclusion about adherence: Kids can't do it alone. When children and youth are given more independent responsibility for illness management, adherence almost invariably declines, as documented below. Yet current definitions and conceptualizations of adherence continue to place the primary responsibility for illness management on the patient starting from early adolescence onward, even while acknowledging that successful adherence reflects collaboration between multiple actors. In part this is due to reliance on theoretical models based on studies of adults, but it also reflects a larger cultural bias that stresses self-reliance. In this chapter we critique this thinking in favor of an approach that focuses on transactions between the relevant actors (patient, family, provider, healthcare system) rather than on the actors themselves, drawing on systems theory and on the transactional model of child development.

The Push for Independent Self-Care

In children and youth with chronic illness, there is a very strong emphasis on promoting independent self-care as soon as possible, and this appears to be equally true among healthcare providers and families. Studies suggest that parents tend to view age 12 as the time that most children should be able to take over many illness-management tasks (Vessey and Miola 1997), and pediatric providers tend to believe that self-management education should begin even earlier (Geenen et al. 2003).

© Springer International Publishing Switzerland 2015

D. D. Schwartz, M. E. Axelrad, *Healthcare Partnerships for Pediatric Adherence,*
SpringerBriefs in Public Health, DOI 10.1007/978-3-319-13668-4_10

There is a lot of evidence that 12 is seen as a "magic number" when it comes to transferring responsibility for illness management from the parent to the child. This is the age that has been found in studies of children with T1D (Wysocki et al. 1996), transplant patients (Shemesh 2004), and asthma (Orrell-Valente et al. 2008). In the study of transplant patients, primary responsibility for medication adherence fell to 30 % of children age 9–10 years, 50 % of children age 11–12, 65–70 % of children age 13–16, and all children 17 and older ($n=81$) (Shemesh 2004). In children with HIV, one descriptive study found that one quarter of patients age 8–18 reported having *full* responsibility for their own medication, and this percentage increased with age (Naar-King et al. 2009).

Twelve is also the age that many writers believe the process should begin for preparing youth for transitioning into adult healthcare. A recent study involving focus groups and interviews with 143 young adults with special health care needs, their family members, and their healthcare providers concluded that preparing youth for transition "should start in childhood or at the time of diagnosis," and that "providers can help to facilitate transition by encouraging families to envision their child's future and promoting medical independence" (Reiss et al. 2005).

Current Practice Recommendations

The influence of these beliefs about fostering "medical independence" has extended into practice recommendations. Current American Academy of Pediatrics (AAP) guidelines recommend that transition planning for youth should begin at the age of 12 years, and possibly even sooner for children with chronic illness (Cooley et al. 2011). Of course, transition planning is different from transfer of responsibility, but the report also recommends that "parents/caregivers must view the youth as the driver in the process and *encourage the youth to assume increasing responsibility for his or her own health care to the fullest extent possible*" [emphasis added].

Underlying this recommendation is the belief that early adolescence is "when youth become developmentally capable of engaging in activities regarding their personal futures." The evidence we reviewed in Chap. 6 would argue against this, however. Adolescents may be intellectually capable of self-care but many lack the social-emotional maturity and self-regulatory capabilities to be successful in daily management of a chronic illness.

The Evidence for Continued Parent Involvement

As the authors of the AAP report note, the guidelines are based on "expert opinion and consensus recommendations" given the lack of sufficient outcome data about transfer of care. However, there are extensive outcome data on premature transfer of responsibility.

Consider children who have received liver and other organ transplants. It is well known that medication nonadherence is the single most common reason for premature graft loss in adolescents (Dobbels et al. 2010; Oliva et al. 2013; Shemesh 2004), and adolescents who have primary responsibility for medication adherence are more likely to be nonadherent than those whose parents are responsible (74 vs. 56% in one study; Simons et al. 2009).

Encouraging transplant patients to be responsible for their medication at an early age would therefore seem ill-advised. However, this is what appears to be occurring at some major pediatric medical centers. A recent article in the Wall Street Journal reported that at Mount Sinai Hospital in New York, parents of liver transplant patients are encouraged "to start letting their children be responsible for taking medication from the age of 10 or so" (Whalen 2014). Unfortunately, such well-meaning attempts to foster greater independence in pediatric patients have the potential to backfire.

The finding that adherence and illness control decline when parent involvement decreases and youth assume more independent responsibility is not specific to pediatric transplant patients. Instead, this is a pattern that has been observed in many diagnostic groups, including asthma (Bender et al. 1998; Duncan et al. 2013; Fiese and Wamboldt 2003), type 1 diabetes (Anderson et al. 2002; Holmes et al 2006; Lewandowski et al. 2007; Lewin et al. 2006; Wysocki et al. 2006), and HIV/AIDS (Mellins et al. 2004; Williams et al. 2006; Naar-King et al. 2009), among other conditions. Moreover, a decline in parent involvement and shift in responsibility can be especially calamitous for youth who are already struggling with adherence (Seiffge-Krenke et al. 2013).

Developmental Readiness

There are benefits to involving youth at the level at which they're ready, although true readiness can be very hard to determine. Moreover, there can be costs to giving youths more responsibility even when they're ready for it. Wysocki et al. (1996) examined self-care responsibility in children ages 5–17 with type 1 diabetes as a function of their assessed psychological maturity. Controlling for age, the children and youth were divided into three groups; youth with:

- Too little responsibility given their assessed maturity
- An appropriate level of responsibility given their assessed maturity
- Too much responsibility given their assessed maturity

The findings are instructive. The group with excessive responsibility did most poorly on every measure, with significantly more hospitalizations than the other two groups, worse adherence and glycemic control, and worse diabetes knowledge. It has been argued that giving children more responsibility results in better disease knowledge, but this did not prove to be the case here, possibly because these youth lacked the parent feedback necessary for effective learning. Having an appropriate level of responsibility resulted in better developed diabetes knowledge than either having too little or too much responsibility, but this came at a cost of having more hospitalizations than youth with less responsibility (although fewer hospitalizations than the excessive responsibility group). Thus, high parental monitoring likely helped keep children with less responsibility out of the ER. (The groups with appropriate and too little responsibility both had good adherence and glycemic control.) Taken together, these findings suggest that maintaining a high level of parent responsibility may be the best short-term strategy with regards to illness control and child safety, although it may not adequately prepare youth for independent self-management.

Barriers to Parent-Child Collaboration

Despite all of the empirical evidence, many healthcare providers remain resistant to the idea of encouraging a high level of parent involvement in youth's chronic illness management (Weissberg-Benchell et al. 1995). There appear to be many reasons for this. Ironically, the movement toward *patient-centered care*, which has transformed adult medicine for the better, may inadvertently reinforce the idea that children need to become independent in self-care as soon as possible. Patient-cantered care emphasizes "individual patient preferences, needs, and values, and ensuring that patient values guide all clinical decisions" (Institute of Medicine 2001). This focus on *individual* preferences and needs is crucial for good adult care but leaves little room for the family involvement so necessary in pediatrics.

From a practical standpoint, there is also the reasonable concern that preparing youth for independent management in later adolescence (i.e., age 16–18) will simply be too late (Cooley et al. 2011). We agree. The question, however, is whether promoting independence from an early age is the best way to prepare youth, an issue we will take up further below.

Complicating the sharing of responsibility between parent and youth is that it is not always clear who is responsible for which aspect of illness management, which creates "diffusion of responsibility" and clear problems for illness management (e.g., Anderson et al. 1990; Dashiff 2003; Martin et al. 2007; Wade et al. 1999). Even worse, in some cases youth simply may not step up to take over the tasks that parents stop doing (Walders et al. 2000). These findings point to a failure or *breakdown of communication* as a likely impediment to successful collaboration (Wysocki 1997)

Family preferences for adolescent independence may also drive the move toward independent self-care (Reiss et al. 2005). Adolescents themselves push for more independence and autonomy as a matter of course, and many parents grow tired of fighting with them over these issues. Adolescence is characterized by increased parent-child conflict and decreased closeness and time spent together (Steinberg and Morris 2001), so maintaining parent involvement can be quite challenging, and healthcare providers may give up hope of seeing their patients and parents get along. Parents may also disengage from illness management if conflict results, despite the fact that this sort of conflict is normal and may actually be an important way that parents and teens renegotiate their relationship around self-care (Holmbeck 1996). Interventions that have focused on teaching families conflict management skills have proved to be an effective way to promote family "teamwork" in children with different chronic illnesses and their parents (Anderson et al. 1999; Duncan et al. 2013).

The Catch-22 of Parent Involvement

Even when parenting is positive and effective, and results in good immediate outcomes, many people remain concerned about the longer term effects on youth development. Specifically, there is the concern that a high level of parent input may foster a level of dependence in youth that would serve them poorly when they make the transition into early adulthood, when they will have to (sooner or later) take over independent management of their care. Indeed, there has recently been a groundswell of popular literature decrying over-parenting and warning parents about smothering their children—so-called "helicopter parenting" (Schiffrin et al. 2013).

Research *does* support the idea that over-involved parenting can have negative effects on development and on adolescents' psychosocial functioning (Barber et al. 1994). Research also indicated that excessive parent control has negative effects on chronic illness outcomes (Butler et al. 2007; Davis et al. 2001; Wiebe et al. 2005). An important caveat is that these studies really document an extreme level of parent involvement and attempted control, and not the more common involvement of most parents.

Nonetheless, this brings us to an apparent Catch-22. Youth independence for adherence can result in better self-efficacy for illness management, yet it entails the substantial risk of declining control that in turn can result in serious complications. In other words, the stakes of independence are higher when a youth has a chronic illness, especially one that is more severe. On the other hand, parent involvement is a key to good illness control, but only if conflict can managed, and it has the potential to delay adolescent development, especially when parent control is excessive.

We believe the solution to this dilemma lies in the distinction noted earlier between *independence* and *autonomy*. As a reminder, being independent means being solely responsible, whereas being autonomous means being self-governing, acting under one's own volition. (Importantly, this distinction is not always made in the literature, and autonomy is often used synonymously with independence—so may the reader beware.) We believe that autonomy support, in the sense of supporting youths' own motivations, choices, and goals *without pushing independent management*, is a cornerstone of collaborative healthcare. In the next chapter we examine the notion of autonomy support in more detail, and present the rudiments of a model of collaborative care.

The Most Vulnerable Patients

Finally, it must be acknowledged that a different set of issues face families who struggle with poverty and often must cope with multiple stressors simultaneously. Maintaining a high level of parent involvement may simply not be realistic for these families (Anderson 2012). This is especially true of single-parent families for whom backup caregivers are unavailable or unreliable. Many parents probably transition responsibility for self-care to their children prematurely because they have no other choice—they have to work. One thinks of recent cases in the news where poor, single mothers had no option but leave their young children unsupervised (in a public park, in a locked car) while they went to work or attended a job interview so as to be able to continue to provide for their families' basic needs (e.g., Shaila Dewan, A job seeker's desperate choice. New York Times June 21, 2014. http://www.nytimes.com/2014/06/22/business/a-job-seekers-desperate-choice.html). It is easy to see how parents struggling to ensure their families' survival would come to rely on their children becoming relatively independent at an early age, including becoming more independent for illness management. However, a parent's necessity should not become a profession's policy, especially when the stakes are as high as in the case of a diabetic child needing to take insulin or a child with HIV needing to take antiretrovirals. Instead, the case must be made for providing external support to these families, possibly through Medicaid or a new provision under the ACA. Enlisting school personnel is also a step in the right direction (NIH Publication No. 13-7739 2013).

Summary and Conclusions

The findings reviewed in this chapter have lead many authors to the conclusion that *family collaboration* around illness management is crucial for the health and well-being of children and youth with chronic illnesses (e.g., Greening et al. 2006; Miller and Drotar 2007; Wysocki et al. 2009). Indeed, the AAP guidelines do also recognize the importance of family collaboration (Cooley et al. 2011). However, there are many barriers to maintaining collaborative efforts. Perhaps foremost of these is the deeply held belief that self-care independence should be the immediate goal.

We are not arguing that self-management is not the *ultimate* goal. Young adults need to be able to independently manage their chronic illness, certainly by the time they are independently managing other aspects of their lives. However, the research evidence is clear that maintaining parent involvement, even into late adolescence, is critically important for helping youth maintain good illness control. *How* that involvement is maintained is a crucial determinant, however, of whether it contributes to or hinders good illness control.

This is also not to say that certain skills deficits cannot be remedied during the time patients' are under pediatric care, and that such efforts are not warranted—they certainly are—but that the benefits are likely to prove limited, at least for higher risk patients whose deficits lie in *using* the skills they have. For problems such as these, an educational and remedial approach (e.g., as recommended by Annunziato et al. 2008) is unlikely to prove very effective (Kahana et al. 2008; see Chap. 4). Instead, when considering the challenges faced by adolescents as a result of normal developmental processes, the evidence again points to parent support and involvement as a critical moderator of risk.

Of course, we recognize that no one is recommending that youth be left fully on their own for illness management, and that the distinction between AAP guidelines and our suggestions is primarily one of emphasis. But we believe that this emphasis is crucial, as the message many patients, parents, and providers seem to have heard is that children must become as independent as possible as soon as possible, and the results have not been good.

References

Anderson BJ. Who forgot? The challenges of family responsibility for adherence in vulnerable pediatric populations. Pediatrics. 2012;129(5):e1324–5.

Anderson BJ, Auslander WF, Jung KC, Miller JP, Santiago JV. Assessing family sharing of diabetes responsibilities. J Pediatr Psychol. 1990;15(4):477–92.

Anderson B, Brackett J, Ho J, Laffel LM. An office-based intervention to maintain parent-adolescent teamwork in diabetes management. Impact on parent involvement, family conflict, and subsequent glycemic control. Diabetes Care 1999;22:713–21.

Anderson BJ, Vangsness L, Connell A, Butler D, Goebel-Fabbri A, Laffel LMB. Family conflict, adherence, and glycaemic control in youth with short duration type 1 diabetes. Diabetic Med. 2002;19:635–42.

Annunziato RA, Emre S, Shneider BL, Dugan CA, Aytaman Y, McKay MM, Shemesh E. Transitioning health care responsibility from caregivers to patient: a pilot study aiming to facilitate medication adherence during this process. Pediatr Transplant. 2008;12:309–15.

Barber BK, Olsen JE, Shagle SC. Associations between parental psychological and behavioral control and youth internalized and externalized behaviors. Child Dev. 1994;65:1120–36.

Bender B, Milgrom H, Rand C, Ackerson L. Psychological factors associated with medication nonadherence in asthmatic children. J Asthma. 1998;35:347–53.

Butler JM, Skinner M, Gelfand D, Berg CA, Wiebe DJ. Maternal parenting style and adjustment in adolescents with type I diabetes. J Pediatr Psychol. 2007;32:1227–37.

Cooley WC, Sagerman PJ, American Academy of Pediatrics, American Academy of Family Physicians, American College of Physicians, Transitions Clinical Report Authoring Group. Supporting the health care transition from adolescence to adulthood in the medical home. Pediatrics. 2011;128:182–200. pmid:21708806.

Dashiff CJ. Self- and dependent-care responsibility of adolescents with IDDM and their parents. J Fam Nurs. 2003;9:166–83.

Davis CL, Delamater AM, Shaw KH, La Greca AM, Eidson MS, Perez-Rodriguez JE, Nemery R. Parenting styles, regimen adherence, and glycemic control in 4- to 10-year-old children with diabetes. J Pediatr Psychol. 2001;26:123–9.

Dewan S. A job seeker's desperate choice. New York Times. 2014 June 21. http://www.nytimes.com/2014/06/22/business/a-job-seekers-desperate-choice.html. Accessed 16 Mar 2015.

Dobbels F, Ruppar T, De Geest S, Decorte A., Van Damme-Lombaerts R, Fine RN. Adherence to the immunosuppressive regimen in pediatric kidney transplant recipients: a systematic review. Pediatr Transplant. 2010;5:603–13.

Duncan CL, Hogan MB, Tien KJ, et al. Efficacy of a parent-youth teamwork intervention to promote adherence in pediatric asthma. J Pediatr Psychol. 2013;38:617–28.

Fiese BH, Wamboldt FS. Tales of pediatric asthma management: family-based strategies related to medical adherence and health care utilization. J Pediatr. 2003;143:457–62.

Geenen SJ, Powers LE, Sells W. Understanding the role of health care providers during the transition of adolescents with disabilities and special health care needs. J Adolesc Health. 2003;32(3):225–33.

Greening L, Stoppelbein L, Reeves CB. A model for promoting adolescents' adherence to treatment for Type 1 diabetes mellitus. Child Heath Care 2006;35:247–67.

Holmbeck G. A model of family relational transformations during the transition to adolescence: parent-adolescent conflict and adaptation. In: Graber J, Brooks-Gunn J, Petersen A, editors. Transitions through adolescence: interpersonal domains and context. Mahwah: Lawrence Erlbaum; 1996.

Holmes CS, Chen R, Streisand R, Marschall DE, Souter S, Swift EE. Predictors of youth diabetes care behaviors and metabolic control: a structural equation modeling approach. J Pediatric Psychol. 2006;31:770–84.

Institute of Medicine. Crossing the quality chasm: a new health system for the 21st century. Washington, DC: The National Academies Press; 2001.

Kahana S, Drotar D, Frazier T. Meta-analysis of psychological interventions to promote adherence to treatment in pediatric chronic health conditions. J Pediatr Psychol 2008;33:590–611.

Lewandowski A, Drotar D. The relationship between parent-reported social support and adherence to medical treatment in families of adolescents with type I diabetes. J Pediatr Psychol. 2007;32:427–36.

Lewin AB, Heidgerken AD, Geffken GR, Williams LB, Stroch EA, Gelfand KM, Silverstein JH. The relations between family factors and metabolic control: the role of diabetes adherence. J Pediatr Psychol. 2006;31:174–83.

Martin S, Elliott-DeSorbo DK, Wolters PL, Toledo-Tamula MA, Roby G, Zeichner S, et al. Patient, caregiver and regimen characteristics associated with adherence to highly active antiretroviral therapy among HIV-infected children and adolescents. Pediatr Infect Dis J. 2007;26:61–7.

Mellins CA, Brackis-Cott E, Dolezal C, Abrams EJ. The role of psychosocial and family factors in adherence to antiretroviral treatment in human immunodeficiency virus-infected children. Pediatr Infect Dis J. 2004;23:1035–41.

Miller VA, Drotar D. Decision-making competence and adherence to treatment in adolescents with diabetes. J Pediatr Psychol. 2007;32:178–88.

Naar-King S, Montepiedra G, Nichols S, PACTG P1042S Team, et al. Allocation of family responsibility for illness management in pedi- atric HIV. J Pediatr Psychol. 2009;34(2):187–94.

Oliva M, Singh TP, Gauvreau K, VanderPluym CJ, Bastardi HJ, Almond CS. Impact of medication non-adherence on survival after pediatric heart transplantation in the USA. J Heart Lung Transplant. 2013;32:881–8.

Orrell-Valente JK, Jarlsberg LG, Hill LG, Cabana MD. At what age do children start taking asthma medicines on their own? Pediatrics. 2008;122:e1186–92.

Reiss JG, Gibson RW, Walker LR. Health care transition: youth, family, and provider perspectives. Pediatrics. 2005;115:112–20.

Schiffrin H, Liss M, Miles-McLean H, Geary KA, Erchull MJ, Tashner T. Helping or hovering? The effects of helicopter parenting on college students' well-being. J Child Fam Stud. 2013;23:548–57.

Seiffge-Krenke I, Laursen B, Dickson DJ, Hartl AC. Declining metabolic control and decreasing parental support among families with adolescents with diabetes: the risk of restrictiveness. J Pediatr Psychol. 2013;38:518–30.

Shemesh E. Non-adherence to medications following pediatric liver transplantation. Pediatr Transplant. 2004;8:600–5.

Simons LE, McCormick ML, Mee LL, Blount RL. Parent and patient perspectives on barriers to medication adherence in adolescent trans- plant recipients. Pediatr Transplant. 2009;13:338–47.

Steinberg LT, Morris AS. Adolescent development. Ann Rev Psychol. 2001;52:83–110.

Vessey JA, Miola ES. Teaching adolescents self-advocacy skills. Pediatr Nurs 1997;23(1):53–6.

Wade SL, Islam S, Holden G, Kruszon-Moran D, Mitchell H. Division of responsibility for asthma management tasks between caregivers and children in the inner city. J Dev Behav Pediatr. 1999;20:93–8.

Walders N, Drotar D, Kercsmar C. The allocation of family responsibility for asthma management tasks in African-American adolescents. J Asthma. 2000;37:89–99.

Weissberg-Benchell J, Glasgow AM, Tynan WD, Wirtz P, Turek J, Ward J. Adolescent diabetes management and mismanagement. Diabetes Care. 1995;18(1):77–82.

Whalen J. New ways to get children to take their medicines: doctors and hospitals get creative to solve a dangerous problem. 2014. http://online.wsj.com/articles/new-ways-to-get-children-to-take-their-medicines-1402064246. Accessed Sept 2014.

Wiebe DJ, Berg CA, Korbel C, Palmer DL, Beveridge RM, Upchurch R, et al. Children's appraisals of maternal involvement in coping with diabetes: enhancing our understanding of adherence, metabolic control, and quality of life across adolescence. J Pediatr Psychol. 2005;30:167–78.

Williams PL, Storm D, Montepiedra G, Nichols S, Kammer B, Sirois PA, et al. Predictors of adherence to antiretroviral medications in children and adolescents with HIV infection. Pediatrics. 2006;118:e1745–57.

Wysocki T. The ten keys to helping your child grow up with diabetes. American Diabetes Association: Alexandria; 1997.

Wysocki T, Taylor A, Hough BS, Linscheid TR, Yeates KO, Naglieri JA. Deviation from developmentally appropriate self-care autonomy: association with diabetes outcomes. Diabetes Care.1996;19(2):119–25.

Wysocki T, Harris MA, Buckloh LM, Wilkinson K, Sadler M, Mauras N, et al. Self-care autonomy and outcomes of intensive therapy or usual care in youth with type 1 diabetes. J Pediatr Psychol. 2006;31:1036–45.

Wysocki T, Nansel TR, Holmbeck GN, et al. Collaborative involvement of primary and secondary caregivers: associations with youths' diabetes outcomes. J Pediatr Psychol. 2009;34:869–81.

Chapter 11
Healthcare Partnerships

Abstract Many authors have concluded that parent involvement and family team-work are key factors in the successful management of pediatric chronic illness, and we agree. However, adherence does not occur solely within the family. Interactions between the family and their healthcare providers are also critical facets of illness management. Yet these interactions can also be fraught with complexities and con-flicts. This chapter expands the idea of family partnerships to the broader one of healthcare partnerships between patients, families, and their providers as the best way to foster and maintain pediatric treatment adherence.

In Chap. 1 we introduced the triadic partnership model developed by De Civita and Dobkin (2004). The basic idea is that adherence behaviors are strongly influenced by transactions between the child, parents, and healthcare providers. However, es-tablishing and maintaining these partnerships is by no means easy.

Perhaps the key challenge in developing healthcare partnerships is finding ways to navigate the challenges posed by adolescence. As discussed previously:

- Early adolescence is the time when many parents and providers begin the shift of responsibility for illness management onto the child
- Adolescents may show cognitive maturity but most lack the social-emotional maturity and self-regulatory capabilities for successful independent management
- Continued parent involvement protects against a decline in illness management and control, provided that parenting is generally positive (authoritative) and con-flict can largely be contained
- Maintaining parent involvement is complicated by the push—from teens, par-ents, and providers—toward ever greater independence
- Adolescents will fight to maintain their sense of independence and autonomy, even in the face of poor or declining illness control

The drive for independence then can be seen as a primary barrier to development of truly collaborative care. A potential way around this problem is to focus instead on fostering patient *autonomy*. Being *autonomy-supportive* does not mean promoting independent decision-making or behavior (unless greater independence reflects the child's goals); instead, it means fostering the youth's goal-attainment and ability to make decisions for him or herself. Since being autonomous "does not preclude

© Springer International Publishing Switzerland 2015   135
D. D. Schwartz, M. E. Axelrad, *Healthcare Partnerships for Pediatric Adherence*,
SpringerBriefs in Public Health, DOI 10.1007/978-3-319-13668-4_11

supportive relationships" (Soenens et al. 2007), it can provide a foundation for collaborative illness management.

Autonomy-Supportive Parenting

Autonomy-supportive parenting actively engages children in decision-making and problem-solving activities, and has been shown to be associated with better adjustment and reduced depression, anxiety, and behavior problems (Padilla-Walker and Nelson 2012). Important aspects of autonomy-supportive parenting include "giving choice, allowing child input into rule making, permitting the expression of ideas, avoiding intrusive behavior" (Padilla-Walker and Nelson 2012), and "allowing children to take an active role in solving their own problems" (Grolnick et al. 1991). Being autonomy-supportive does not preclude providing guidance if requested.

It also does not preclude parental limit-setting. As suggested by Soenens et al. (2007), "when enforcing rules or setting limits (autonomy-supportive parents] would still be interested in the child's perspective and empathic with contrary feelings.... That is, they would not deny a child's 'voice,' even when there is no 'choice.'" In this respect, autonomy-supportive parenting is congruent with authoritative parenting (Chap. 7), and in fact the two terms are often used synonymously in different studies.

In our view, many parents and providers attempt to promote youths' *independence* where they should instead be promoting youth *autonomy*. Not only does greater youth independence for illness management typically result in poorer illness control, as documented above, but attempts to push youth to be more independent might themselves be perceived as coercive and result in increased conflict, which can result in even greater deterioration in self-care (miscarried helping).

These views on adolescent development are in contrast to *separation–individuation* theory (Blos 1979), which posits that it is developmentally important for youth to begin to separate themselves physically and emotionally from their parents, and take increasing responsibility for themselves without relying on parental support. While some theorists continue to see separation as necessary to healthy development, others note that it can have significant costs (Soenens et al. 2007). Parent attempts to promote independence might be perceived by some youth as attempt to "break ties with them" (Grolnick et al. 1997), whereas autonomy support encourages growth within the context of a continued, though changing, relationship. In this sense, autonomy support is quite similar to the notion of *interdependence* first developed by Baumrind (1987). As noted by Anderson et al. (2000), interdependence

is consistent with developmental theories that conceptualize the major task of the adolescent period as movement away from dependence on the family, not toward independence, but rather toward interdependence. Interdependence does not require adolescents to distance themselves emotionally from parents, but rather requires a reorganization in which family members renegotiate and redistribute responsibilities and obligations. (p. 360)

There is good evidence that autonomy-supportive parenting results in better adherence, illness control, parent-child relations, and youth adjustment, above and beyond the copious literature showing positive effects of parental involvement and negative effects of family conflict. Anderson and colleagues (Anderson et al. 1999) developed a family teamwork intervention for young adolescents with type 1 diabetes and their parents focused on sustaining parent involvement and preventing or reducing conflict. The intervention was developed with the idea of fostering interdependence, and included a module in which the parent and child worked together to negotiate a plan to share responsibility for diabetes management. Thus, the intervention supported youth autonomy within the context of family teamwork. The intervention prevented the deterioration in parent involvement typically seen in this age group and reduced the likelihood of parent-child conflict, compared to an attention control group. The teamwork group also had better blood glucose monitoring, which was associated with lower A1c.

More recently, Duncan et al. (2013) adapted the teamwork intervention for children with asthma and their parents. Results were similar, with the teamwork group showing lower parent-child conflict, higher adherence, and better asthma control. In contrast to Anderson et al. however, the intervention used a fading procedure, whereby teens would move to levels of greater independence (i.e., reduced parent monitoring) based on achieving specified adherence goals. However, the specific effect of using this fading system was unclear.

There is also some evidence that autonomy supportive parenting may also be beneficial for adherence in younger children. In an observational study of children aged 2–8 years with type 1 diabetes and their mothers, Chisholm and colleagues (2010) found that children whose mothers involved them in decision-making during a diabetes-related problem-solving task and used "gentle guidance" (e.g., suggestions) rather than commands had better adherence to dietary restrictions and showed a trend for better glycemic control. They concluded that "treatment adherence and health are optimized when children are offered developmentally sensitive opportunities to participate in decisions about their diabetes care," and that "maternal statements which are 'autonomy supportive' and which promote shared responsibility are key features of children's treatment cooperation." Consistent with this, Hanna and Guthrie (2003) found that adolescent autonomy in diabetes decision-making but *not* in diabetes functioning (i.e., independent task completion) was significantly correlated with metabolic control.

Autonomy-Supportive Healthcare

...promoting autonomy among patients, which is advocated within biomedical ethics, does not refer to merely leaving them alone to decide and act for themselves. Rather, it means encouraging them to make choices about how to behave, providing them with the information they need for making the choices, and respecting the choices they make. (Deci and Ryan 2012)

Healthcare providers can also be autonomy-supportive rather than independence-promoting. As Deci and Ryan (2012) suggest, promoting health behavior change involves "both reliance on providers *and* support for autonomy" (emphasis added). The basic idea of being autonomy-supportive is that it is the patient (and often his/her family) who is the ultimate decision-maker. As discussed above, a person can be pushed to be independent before he is ready. An extreme example would be the teenager who is kicked out of his parents' house. His independence would not be the result of autonomous action but instead something forced on him. As Schiffrin et al. (2013) note, "It is possible for parents [or healthcare providers] who intend to promote autonomy to actually be forcing their child toward independence when the child desires more guidance and support."

Well-meaning practitioners often use incentives and contingencies to motivate their patients, or they may refer to their own authority as health experts to elicit change (Ryan et al. 2008). Unfortunately, these attempts can be perceived by patients and families as subtle forms of control, which can undermine provider efforts by undermining patients' sense of autonomy. Even provision of health-related information can backfire if patients perceive the information as coercive in some manner (e.g., "scare tactics"). Deci and Ryan (2012) suggest the importance of providing health information in a consciously dispassionate way so that it is not perceived as coercive, and instead is presented as a means of enhancing the patient's ability to make fully informed choices. As they note, "it is all-too-easy for patients to view healthcare professionals as authorities and to interpret their words as controlling," even when this is not the provider's intent.

> For example, practitioners might say to their patients who smoke cigarettes: "As your provider, I would like to advise you that it is important for your health to try giving up smoking cigarettes. I understand that using tobacco can help you feel better at times and that breaking the tobacco habit can be very difficult. I also believe that whether or not you do try to stop is wholly your choice. I merely want to say that I think it would be useful for you to give this serious consideration and to make a choice about whether to continue smoking or to try stopping. I would respect whichever option you chose."—Deci and Ryan 2012.

Of course, some patients express a preference for a directive approach (Drotar et al. 2010; Resnicow and McMaster 2012). In fact, this is exactly what many patients come to a health expert for. In this case, being directive—telling a patient what she needs to do—is also autonomy-supportive, in that it reflects the patient's expressed desire (Deci and Ryan 2012).

> The opposite of being autonomy supportive is being controlling."—Deci and Ryan 2012

There is some direct evidence for the effectiveness of an autonomy-supportive approach among providers. For example, Williams et al. (1998) found that patients' perception of healthcare providers autonomy support was related to increased motivation, feelings of competence, and significant improvement in glycemic control. Other authors have suggested that autonomy support is a critical aspect of developing a collaborative approach to pediatric chronic illness care (Delamater 2006; Drotar et al. 2010).

Provider-Patient Communication is the Key to Building and Maintaining Partnerships

In Chap. 9, we discussed how physician communication styles are believed to be a major contributor to health disparities and nonadherent behaviors in racial/ethnic minorities. Of course, provider-patient communication is also critically important for promoting adherence in non-minority patients as well (Zolnierek and DiMatteo 2009). Unfortunately, studies have documented poor provider-patient communication in many settings (Brown and Bussell 2011). Poor communication contributes to adherence difficulties (Drotar 2009; Levetown 2008), whereas improving communication also improves adherence (Zolnierek and DiMatteo 2009).

Communication and other interpersonal factors powerfully influence the development of a working therapeutic relationship between healthcare providers and families, and the quality of this relationship determines to a large degree than whether providers will be effective in promoting good illness management in their patients. For example, many children and their parents report feeling "shamed and blamed" by physicians when their illness control declines (Ginsburg et al. 2005; Wolpert and Anderson 2001), which can further contribute to suboptimal adherence (Anderson and Coyne 1991), and may make families more reluctant to come in for follow-up care (Bodenlos et al. 2007). Communication is likely to be especially important when problematic adherence is being driven by differences between providers and patients (and their families) in their views of the illness or its treatment (De Civita and Dobkin 2004).

It is also important to acknowledge how difficult it can be for patients and families to adhere to every aspect of complex medical regimens all the time (Drotar et al. 2010), and taking an understanding, non-judgmental approach to talking about adherence can open the door to having practical and honest conversations about what is realistic for each family (Wolpert and Anderson 2001). Rather than asking some variation of, "You are taking all of your medications, right?" providers may want to try saying, "I know it can be hard to take all of your medications all of the time and most people don't follow the prescription perfectly. Tell me about how it's going for you. How many doses do you think you took this week and how many were missed?"

The responses providers give to these questions are just as important as asking the questions. Responding with, "Well, missing even one dose per week raises your risk of X problem" will likely be less effective than accepting and reinforcing what the patient *has* done, and working together to set a goal for a small increase over the upcoming week (e.g., adding in one more dose per day at a time that is convenient). When talking to patients about prescriptions and treatment recommendations, it is useful to ask families about their unique preferences, beliefs, adherence barriers, and adherence facilitators, and to make treatment recommendations and prescriptions that are realistic in the context of what you have learned.

Making Communication More Autonomy-Supportive Deci and Ryan (2012) make the point that "it is all-too-easy for patients to view healthcare professionals as authorities and to interpret their words as controlling"—call this the implicit bias of the patient. Information that is presented in a way that acknowledges the difficulty of the action or decision (e.g., to begin exercising or quit smoking), and that conveys respect for the patient's ultimate decision (whatever it may be), is likely to be more effective (because it is autonomy-supportive) than communications that make patients feel they are being controlled.

To this end, Deci and Ryan suggest the importance of providing health information in a dispassionate way, so that it is non-coercive and can be used by the family to make fully informed choices; impassioned statements (e.g., "If you don't improve your blood sugar control you'll die an early death") tend to be perceived as subtle or not so subtle forms of attempted control. This point is captured nicely in the title of a recent article on adherence in pediatric cancer: "Do As I Say or Die: Compliance in Adolescents With Cancer" (Windebank and Spinetta 2008). It should be noted that one of the authors' primary conclusions is for the need to improve communication as a way of fostering teens' involvement in their own medical care.

Comprehensive suggestions for physician training in communication skills is provided in Chap. 9. Here we just want to reiterate and highlight a few key points. To foster good communication skills, training programs should teach or include a focus on: effective listening skills (Drotar et al. 2010), collaborative decision-making (Charles et al. 1997; Drotar et al. 2010), autonomy support (Deci and Ryan 2012), and cultural competence (Burgess et al. 2007), with the ultimate goal of building effective partnerships with families.

Patient-Parent-Provider Teamwork: The Healthcare Partnership or Therapeutic Triad

Although the lion's share of decision-making concerning the day-to-day management of chronic conditions is done by parents and children, providers may also be involved in these decisions, especially if families request their advice.—Drotar et al. 2010

The key components to developing a healthcare partnership between children, their parents, and their healthcare providers are:

- Positive relationships (warmth and acceptance between parent and child; a therapeutic alliance between provider and family (Orlinsky et al. 2004)
- An explicit understanding/agreement regarding the need for three-way collaboration
- Effective communication between all parties
- Perceived helpfulness and autonomy support
- Parent involvement (with conflict management as needed)
- Flexibility to respond to changes (in disease course, development, family situation)

From the start, it will be important for the provider to stress that her relationship with the family is (or should be) a collaborative one, that they should work on building an alliance together, and that the provider's role will be to provide the family with her medical expertise so that they can use it to make informed decisions, with or without her input, as they decide. After all, families *are* the primary decision-makers about day-to-day care, whatever the provider may want (Drotar et al. 2010).

Perhaps even more importantly, providers should encourage parents and children to work together and discuss any issues related to illness management that arise (Drotar et al. 2010). One way to do this would be to suggest that families schedule a "family meeting" every week for open discuss of any health-related issues anyone wants to bring to the table (Wysocki 1997). Meetings should have clear ground rules everyone agrees to beforehand, such as:

- Anyone can set agenda items
- Make topic clear and stay on topic
- Give one person the floor at a time
- Limit time spent on any topic (10–15 min)
- Emphasize calm communication and problem-solving
- If someone gets upset, have everyone take a short break
- Use meetings to come up with questions/concern to bring to the next clinic visit

The provider can ask about meetings during follow-up visits; if the family reports a lot of conflict, referral to a behavioral health specialist might prove helpful.

Triadic involvement in decision-making is more complex. Healthcare providers make initial decisions about treatment based on best practice guidelines (or that is the hope, anyway) and the available empirical evidence, and then expect that their patients and families will follow this advice. Collaborative decision-making, when it is engaged in, typically only happens after the initial treatment regimen is set (Drotar et al. 2010). This may be an unavoidable consequence of the complexities of modern medical management, but it can be off-putting for families who feel left out from the start. Taking time to explain the reasons behind initial medical decisions is a tenet of good patient-centered care—when working with families, it is important to involve both child and parent in the discussion. During follow-up visits, asking the patient and parent about quality of life issues is of paramount importance, as is asking about any treatment-related difficulties.

Providers can also foster collaborative teamwork by involving the child in developmentally appropriate ways regardless of age. Even very young children may have questions or misconceptions about the disease or its treatment. Studies suggest that children and adolescents feel that they are often not spoken to or listened to in pediatric visits, and they are rarely involved in decisions about their healthcare; moreover, parents sometimes shut down children's communication during visits (Tates and Meeuwesen 2000). Healthcare providers should find ways to involve the child and give her a voice; when children do participate, their input can often be valuable (Garth et al. 2009). Listening to a child's input does not necessarily mean allowing her to dictate what decisions are made, however; as suggested by Soenen's et al. (2007), providers do not need to "deny a child's 'voice,' even when there is no 'choice.'" In the end, most final decisions are made by parents (Dunst and Paget 1991), although with older teens this may not always be the case.

Developing a Shared Model of Illness

In a classic paper, Kleinman and colleagues (1978) introduced a clinical method for working with patients to develop a shared model of illness. They suggested that clinicians first ask five questions to assess a patient's conceptualization of an illness, and an additional three questions to determine its psychosocial and cultural meaning to the patient:

- What do you think has caused your problem?
- Why do you think it started when it did?
- What do you think your sickness does to you? How does it work?
- How severe is your sickness? Will it have a short or long course?
- What kind of treatment do you think you should receive?
- What are the most important results you hope to receive from this treatment?
- What are the chief problems your sickness has caused for you?
- What do you fear most about your sickness?

After eliciting the patient's model through these questions, the physician is advised to "articulate the doctor's model in simple and direct terms for each of the five major issues of clinical concern." He then should compare both models openly, "pointing out discrepancies in the two views of clinical reality." Finally, the clinician "actively negotiates with the patient, *as a therapeutic ally*, about treatment and expected outcomes."

Kleinman et al.'s procedure was designed to explore *cultural* differences in explanatory models of disease and illness, but it is a useful model for within-culture comparisons as well. As noted by De Civita and Dobkin (2004), development of a collaborative effort among patients, parents, and healthcare providers "may be impeded when there are clashes of different views and discrepant beliefs about illness and treatment within the caregiver-child-provider relationship." As noted earlier, places whether patients and providers may not see eye to eye include the following:

- The patient is concerned about managing *illness* whereas the provider is concerned about managing the *disease*
- The patient and provider have different goals (e.g., maintaining quality of life versus maintaining physiological homeostasis)
- The patient and provider disagree about the best type of treatment (e.g., homeopathy)
- The patient and provider disagree about whether the patient even has a disease
- The patient may not fully trust the provider, especially if they are from different socioeconomic or racial/ethnic backgrounds

Providers who are unaware of these differences, or who do not treat them respectfully, will have a hard time facilitating any sort of behavior change. One could do worse than use Kleinman et al.'s general procedure to discover more about the patient's and parent's understanding of the illness and its meaning to them.

Of course, it is equally important for patients to communicate to their healthcare providers, who are otherwise forced to "operate in the dark." Yet here too provider communication is critical to establish the trust needed for patients to feel comfortable to share their concerns, beliefs, and practices. For example, many patients and their parents do not tell medical professionals about the home remedies they may be using in addition to (or in lieu of) the prescribed treatment regimen, because they know that, in general, medical professionals are dismissive of alternative treatments. This is not to say that empirically-minded professionals should be accepting of alternative treatments per se, but they should create an environment in which the patient is comfortable enough to discuss treatment issues without feeling judged.

Figure 11.1 shows how the therapeutic triad might vary based on different relationships between the three partners. Communication (a) and having a strong shared model (b) is what ties each node together; conflict (c) can push them apart. The overlap between circles is meant to represent alliance strength, which in turn can be taken as an indirect measure of the degree to which the partners have a shared model of illness. (Whether alliance strength and model overlap do in fact correlate is a question for future research.)

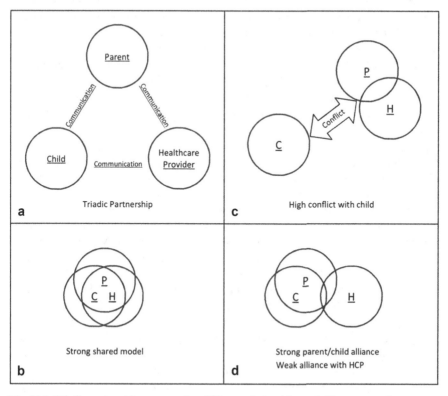

Fig. 11.1 Triadic partnerships representing different relationships and alliance strengths

Coordination of Care

Pediatricians and other primary care providers also act as the "point person" for families, setting them up with needed resources and care that falls outside of the therapeutic triad. Where possible, collaborating with a social worker can make the difference for families who are having trouble getting insurance coverage or accessing other resources. For patients with more entrenched adherence difficulties, or nonadherence in the context of psychosocial or family factors, referral to a pediatric psychologist or behavioral health specialist may be necessary to have any chance of fostering behavioral change. We close this chapter with a brief discussion of the role psychologists can play in helping children and their families manage a chronic illness.

The Role of Psychologists

Psychologists with training in behavioral health play a critical role in the delivery of adherence promotion interventions in pediatric health care. Traditionally, pediatric patients have been referred to psychologists only when they presented with comorbid psychological concerns such as depression, or when adherence problems had become severe and entrenched, or when family functioning declined to the degree that the medical provider felt unable to do more than watch the disaster unfold. However, we will also argue that there is room for psychologists to take an expanded role in adherence promotion, specifically with regards to screening and assessment, and development of interventions at different levels of need.

Although many new protocols have been developed that involve medical providers in delivering adherence promotion interventions, the majority of established behavioral interventions have been designed for and delivered by clinical psychologists, psychology trainees, clinical social workers, and other mental health professionals with extensive training in behavioral health. Nine times out of ten, adherence issues are *behavioral* issues, which is almost certainly why behavioral interventions have the strongest empirical support.

Pediatric psychologists are especially well-suited to assess the specific barriers and facilitators of adherence that an individual and family are experiencing, and to provide tailored behavioral interventions (Guilfoyle et al. 2013; Moser et al. 2014). Examples of practical intervention approaches in the behavioral specialist's "toolbox" include pill-swallowing training to address mechanical or psychological difficulties with medication administration (Hankinson and Slifer 2013), adherence-related goal-setting and problem-solving (Guilfoyle et al. 2013), using electronic monitoring technology as a therapy tool (Herzer et al. 2012), and individual and family-based therapies to address family teamwork and parenting practices to facilitate adherence (Wu and Hommel 2014). Psychologists are also best situated to be able to draw upon the effective multi-component interventions reported here (Wu and Hommel 2014).

The importance of psychologists and other behavioral health specialists to adherence promotion is increasingly being recognized. For example, the ADA's current treatment guidelines for children and youth with type 1 diabetes (American Diabetes Association 2014) recommend incorporating psychological assessment and treatment into routine care and suggest "collaborative care interventions and use of a team approach" when working with mental health professionals.

Psychologists also have a pivotal role in the development and dissemination of universal and low-intensity interventions that can be implemented by others. Anderson et al.'s (1999) teamwork intervention is a model for this sort of work, as it was designed to be used by clinical staff (physicians, nurses, even paraprofessionals) with minimal behavioral training in the course of routine care. Some further examples are presented in the last chapter, when we describe a preliminary model for providing both prevention and intervention services focused on adherence at three different levels of assessed risk and need (cf. Kazak 2006).

Summary and Conclusions

In an ACO [accountable care organization] model, it may not be unreasonable to reward both parents and children with the disease for their work as partners with the medical team to achieve optimal outcomes.—Stark 2013

Managing a child's chronic medical condition is a complex endeavor that requires the coordinated efforts of patients, parents, and healthcare providers. The need for developing healthcare partnerships is motivated by extensive research showing that it is dangerous for youth with chronic illness to "go it alone." Even when youth and their families want to take on this risk, it should be kept in mind that from a public health perspective, the costs of adolescent independence to society as well as to the individual patient can be huge. Autonomy-support is necessary in many instances to gain adolescent cooperation and acceptance of receiving help, without threatening (and indeed fostering) age-appropriate development.

Communication is the key to building and maintaining these partnerships. Communication is necessary for assessing adherence, resolving conflict, and engaging families in decision-making. Declines in adherence are often the direct result of communication breakdowns (Wysocki 1997). Communication also fosters the development of a shared model of illness, without which patients, families, and providers may find themselves working at cross purposes, although without good communication they would never know it.

The healthcare partnership we have described here is based on the notion of the therapeutic triad of De Civita and Dobkin (2004), but importantly it allows for the inclusion of additional members of the partnership team. In particular, it is often necessary to include a psychologist with expertise in behavioral health to help manage clinical issues that have become too big for the triad to manage effectively.

It follows from the arguments above that the most successful interventions for adherence problems are likely be those with a focus on strengthening the relationships between the different healthcare partners. There is a growing evidence base in support of this hypothesis, but especially given the complexities involved in three-way interactions, this remains an important area for future research.

References

American Diabetes Association. Standards of medical care in diabetes—2014. Diabetes Care. 2014;37(1):14–80.

Anderson BJ, Coyne JC. "Miscarried helping" in the interactions between chronically ill children and their parents. In: Johnson JH, Johnson SB, editors. Advances in child health psychology. Gainesville: University of Florida Press; 1991. pp. 167–77.

Anderson B, Brackett J, Ho J, Laffel LM. An office-based intervention to maintain parent-adolescent teamwork in diabetes management. Impact on parent involvement, family conflict, and subsequent glycemic control. Diabetes Care. 1999;22:713–21.

Anderson B, Brackett J, Ho J, Laffel L. An intervention to promote family teamwork in diabetes management tasks: relationships among parental involvement, adherence to blood glucose monitoring, and glycemic control in young adolescents with type 1 diabetes. In: Drotar D, editor. Promoting adherence to medical treatment in chronic childhood illness: concepts, methods, and interventions. New Jersey: Lawrence Erlbaum; 2000. pp. 347–66.

Baumrind D. A developmental perspective on adolescent risk taking in contemporary America. New Dir Child Adolesc Dev. 1987;1987(37):93–125.

Blos P. The adolescent passage. Madison: International Universities Press; 1979.

Bodenlos J, Grothe K, Whitehead D, Konkle-Parker D, Jones G, Brantley P. Attitudes toward health care providers and appointment attendance in HIV/AIDS patients. J Assoc Nurses AIDS Care. 2007;18:65–73.

Brown MT, Bussell JK. Medication adherence: WHO cares. Mayo Clin Proc. 2011;86(4):304–14.

Burgess D, van Ryn M, Dovidio J, Saha S. Reducing racial bias among health care providers: lessons from social-cognitive psychology. J Gen Intern Med. 2007;22(6):882–7.

Charles C, Gafni A, Whelan T. Shared decision-making in the medical encounter: what does it mean? (or it takes at least two to tango). Soc Sci Med. 1997;44(5):681–92.

Chisholm V, Atkinson L, Donaldson C, Noyes K, Payne A, Kelnar C. Maternal communication style, problem-solving and dietary adherence in young children with type 1 diabetes. Clin Child Psychol Psychiatry. 2011;16(3):443–58.

De Civita M, Dobkin PL. Pediatric adherence as a multidimensional and dynamic construct, involving a triadic partnership. J Pediatr Psychol. 2004;29:157–69.

Deci EL, Ryan RM. Self-determination theory in health care and its relations to motivational interviewing: a few comments. Int J Behav Nutr Phys Act. 2012;9:24.

Delamater AM. Improving patient adherence. Clin Diabetes. 2006;24:71–7.

Drotar D. Physician behavior in the care of pediatric chronic illness: association with health outcomes and treatment adherence. J Dev Behav Pediatr. 2009;30:246–54.

Drotar D, Crawford P, Bonner M. Collaborative decision making and treatment adherence promotion in the management of pediatric chronic illness. Patient Intell. 2010;2:1–7.

Duncan CL, Hogan MB, Tien KJ, Portnoy J. Efficacy of a parent-youth teamwork intervention to promote adherence in pediatric asthma. J Pediatr Psychol. 2013;38:617–28.

Dunst C, Paget K. Parent–professional partnerships and family empowerment. In: Fine M, editor. Collaboration with parents of exceptional children. Brandon: Clinical Psychology Publishing Company; 1991. pp. 25–44.

Garth B, Murphy GC, Reddihough DS. Perceptions of participation: child patients with a disability in the doctor–parent–child partnership. Patient Educ Couns. 2009;74:45–52.

Ginsburg KR, Howe CJ, Jawad AF, et al. Parents' perceptions of factors that affect successful diabetes management for their children. Pediatrics. 2005;116:1095–104.

Grolnick WS, Ryan RM, Deci EL. Inner resources for school achievement: motivational mediators of children's perceptions of their parents. J Educ Psychol. 1991;83:508–17.

Grolnick WS, Ryan RM, Deci EL. Internalization in the family: the self-determination perspective. In: Grusec JE, Kuczynski L, editors. Parenting and children's internalization of values. NY: Wiley; 1997.

Guilfoyle SM, Follansbee-Junger K, Modi AC. Development and preliminary implementation of a psychosocial service into standard medical care for pediatric epilepsy. Clin Pract Pediatr Psychol. 2013;1:276–88.

Hankinson JC, Slifer KJ. Behavioral treatments to improve pill swallowing and adherence in an adolescent with renal and connective tissue diseases. Clinical Practice in Pediatric Psychology 2013; 1(3): 227–234.

Hanna KM, Guthrie D. Adolescents' behavioral autonomy related to diabetes management and adolescent activities/rules. Diabetes Educ. 2003;29(2):283–91.

Herzer M, Ramey C, Rohan J, Cortina S. Incorporating electronic monitoring feedback into clinical care: a novel and promising adherence promotion approach. Clin Child Psychol Psychiatry. 2012;17:505–18.

Kazak AE. Pediatric Psychosocial Preventative Health Model (PPPHM): research, practice and collaboration in pediatric family systems medicine. Fam Syst Health. 2006;24:381–95.

Kleinman AM, Eisenberg L, Good B. Culture, illness, and care. Clinical lessons from anthropological and cross-cultural research. Ann Intern Med. 1978;88:251–8.

Levetown M, The Committee on Bioethics. Communicating with children and families: from everyday interactions to skill in conveying distressing information. Pediatrics. 2008;121:e1441–60.

Moser NL, Plante WA, LeLeiko NS, Lobato DJ. Integrating behavioral health services into pediatric gastroenterology: a model of an integrated health care program. Clin Pract Pediatr Psychol. 2014;2:1–12.

Orlinsky DE, Ronnestad MH, Willutski U. Fifty years of psychotherapy process-outcome research: continuity and change. In: Lambert MJ, editor. Handbook of psychotherapy and behaviour change. 5th ed. New York: John Wiley & Sons; 2004.

Padilla-Walker LM, Nelson LJ. Black Hawk Down? Establishing helicopter parenting as a distinct construct from other forms of parental control during emerging adulthood. J Adolesc. 2012;35:1177–90.

Resnicow K, McMaster F. Motivational interviewing: moving from why to how with autonomy support. Int J Behav Nutr Phys Act. 2012;9:19.

Ryan RM, Patrick H, Deci EL, Williams GC. Facilitating health behaviour change and its maintenance: interventions based on self-determination theory. Eur Health Psychol. 2008;10:2–5.

Schiffrin H, Liss M, Miles-McLean H, Geary KA, Erchull MJ, Tashner T. Helping or hovering? The effects of helicopter parenting on college students' well-being. J Child Fam Stud. 2013;23:548–57.

Soenens B, Vansteenkiste M, Lens W, Luyckx K, Goossens L, Beyers W, Ryan RM. Conceptualizing parental autonomy support: adolescent perceptions of promotion of independence versus promotion of volitional functioning. Dev Psychol. 2007;43:633–46.

Stark L. Introduction to the special issue on adherence in pediatric medical conditions. J Pediatr Psychol. 2013;38:589–94.

Tates K, Meeuwesen L. 'Let mum have her say': turn taking in doctor-parent-child communication. Patient Educ Couns. 2000;40:151–62.

Williams GC, Freedman ZR, Deci EL. Supporting autonomy to motivate patients with diabetes for glucose control. Diabetes Care. 1998;21:1644–51.

Windebank KP, Spinetta JJ. Do as i say or die: compliance in adolescents with cancer. Pediatr Blood Cancer. 2008;50:1099–100.

Wolpert HA, Anderson BJ. Management of diabetes: are doctors framing the benefits from the wrong perspective? BMJ. 2001;323:994–6.

Wu YP, Hommel KA. Using technology to assess and promote adherence to medical regimens in pediatric chronic illness. J Pediatr. 2014;164(4):922–7.

Wysocki T. The ten keys to helping your child grow up with diabetes. Alexandria: American Diabetes Association; 1997.

Zolnierek KBH, DiMatteo MR. Physician communication and patient adherence to treatment: a meta-analysis. Med Care. 2009;47:826–34.

Part III
Looking Ahead

A Comprehensive Behavioral Health Model for Promoting Pediatric Adherence

Chapter 12
Screening for Nonadherence in Pediatric Patients

Abstract Screening provides the foundation for all subsequent clinical decision making. Moreover, it makes possible a preventive approach, which we argue is critical to improving the health and well-being of children. This chapter discusses the rationale for screening, lays out a blueprint for developing a psychosocial screening program, and describes our experience in implementing a screening program in a busy pediatric hospital. We focus primarily on children and youth with type 1 diabetes, as this has been an active area of our research. The chapter also links to tools clinicians can use to screen their patients, and provides guidance in their use specifically written for professionals who lack training in psychology. A version of Kazak's Pediatric Psychosocial Preventive Health Model is presented as a guide for clinical decision-making.

Introduction

It has been suggested that physicians are at no better than chance levels when identifying or predicting non-adherence in their patients (Phillips et al. 2011). Having a reliable and valid, evidence-based method for assessing for nonadherence is therefore critical for identifying patients who need additional support or intervention. It is equally important to assess psychosocial factors known to contribute to nonadherence.

How does one screen for nonadherence? Most obviously, the physician can look for clinical signs of poor or declining illness control that are not explained by other variables. For example, most incidents of DKA in patients with established diabetes (i.e., not newly-diagnosed) are attributable to a small set of factors: illness (such as flu), pump malfunction (if the patient is on an insulin pump), and not taking insulin (nonadherence). DKA in the absence of the first two factors is therefore a reasonably reliable sign of nonadherence (Wolfsdorf et al. 2009).

© Springer International Publishing Switzerland 2015
D. D. Schwartz, M. E. Axelrad, *Healthcare Partnerships for Pediatric Adherence,*
SpringerBriefs in Public Health, DOI 10.1007/978-3-319-13668-4_12

However, such cases are probably the exception, not the rule. What if the same diabetes patient has an increase in A1c from 8 to 9 %? Is this a sign of nonadherence, or does it reflect any number of other factors? A second point can also be made about this example. As is well known, DKA can be life-threatening. Is there any way to *predict* who might be at heightened risk for DKA, so that preventive measures might be taken?

Screening as we operationalize it here has two main goals. First, *risk screening* that occurs at diagnosis (or soon thereafter) has the goal of identifying patients at risk for nonadherence and poor illness control. The idea is to predict who might be at heightened risk, so that preventive measures might be taken. Risk screening allows for potential problems to be addressed before they have become entrenched or severe, and thus will be more amenable to intervention (Gates 2001; Modi et al. 2013).

Second *surveillance screening* of established patients is critical to identify who might be nonadherent or struggling with other issues that can affect adherence, such as depression. Again, earlier identification is better. Surveillance screening is justified because (1) problems are not always identified at onset, (2) factors that influence a child's functioning are dynamic and change over time—these include development, changes within the family, and changes in disease course, among others (De Civita and Dobkins 2004), and (3) problems often do not develop until later on. For example, in youth with diabetes, problems with depression and anxiety are more likely in the second year following diagnosis (Grey et al. 1995), and it often takes a few years for adherence problems to emerge (Kovacs et al. 1992), probably because over time children get tired of managing an illness day in and out. Another factor for patients diagnosed in early-middle childhood is that adherence is likely to decline with onset of puberty (Chap. 6). It has recently been suggested that surveillance screening should be a part of children's ongoing medical care (Stark 2013).

The Importance of Prevention

Nonadherent behaviors, once established, are very hard to treat or reverse (Anderson et al. 2002). Moreover, negative health outcomes tend to snowball once patterns of nonadherence become set. Conversely, development of good habits of adherence early in the course of an illness can protect against later negative health outcomes (Writing Team for the Diabetes Control and Complications Trial/Epidemiology of Diabetes Interventions and Complications Research Group 2003). Thus, a key aspect to improving the health and well-being of children and adolescents and preventing or reducing serious complications of chronic illness is to focus on prevention of nonadherence, or early intervention for nonadherent behaviors that have not yet had time to become fully entrenched. In recognition of this, the recently passed Affordable Care Act places substantial emphasis on increasing access to preventive services (Kocher et al. 2010). As Koh and Sibelius (2010) conclude, "Moving prevention toward the mainstream of health may well be one of the most lasting legacies of this landmark legislation." Screening—especially risk screening near the time of diagnosis—is critical for any efforts at preventive intervention.

Criteria for Effective Screening

Morrison (1992, 1998) suggested a number of important criteria for screening. These include:

1. Is the problem of sufficient concern and is prevalence high enough to warrant screening?
2. Can problems or risk for problems be detected at screening?
3. Are there reliable (sensitive and specific) methods for screening?
4. Is screening feasible?
5. Is screening acceptable to patients and their families?
6. Is there intervention for identified problems?

Each of these factors is addressed in turn below.

Is the problem of sufficient concern? As noted in Chap. 1, nonadherence can have a dramatic effect on the lives of individual patients, causing or contributing to serious complications of illness, both acute and long-term. Nonadherence also has a substantial impact on the health of populations throughout the world (Sabate 2003). Prevalence rates suggest that some degree of nonadherence is more common than not.

Psychosocial sequelae of illness also have dramatic effects on the health and well-being of individuals and populations. Taking just depression as an example, current guidelines of the US Preventive Services Task Force (2009) note that depression in youth "is a disabling condition that is associated with serious long-term morbidities and risk of suicide. However, the majority of depressed youth are undiagnosed and untreated." Depression is nearly twice as common in youth with diabetes, and it is associated with nonadherence and poor illness control (Hood et al. 2006).

Can problems or risk of problems be detected at diagnosis? Are there reliable screening tools? Problems with adapting to a chronic illness often occur at diagnosis. Nearly a third of children develop an adjustment disorder at disease diagnosis (Cameron et al. 2007). While adjustment problems tend to resolve over the first year, children who experience them are at greater risk for subsequent problems with depression and anxiety (Grey et al. 1995). Acute stress symptoms at disease diagnosis are also elevated for a number of conditions (e.g., Cline et al. 2011) and predict later risk for PTSD.

A number of approaches have been developed for assessing risk at disease diagnosis. Kazak et al. (2001) developed the Psychosocial Assessment Tool (PAT) for screening children diagnosed with cancer. The measure was able to reliably categorize risk according to a public health framework at three levels: Universal, Targeted, and Clinical (Fig. 12.1). *Universal* patients had adequate resources for coping, *Targeted* patients had identified risk factors, and *Clinical* patients had significant current psychosocial stressors. In follow-up work Kazak et al. 2003, 2011;

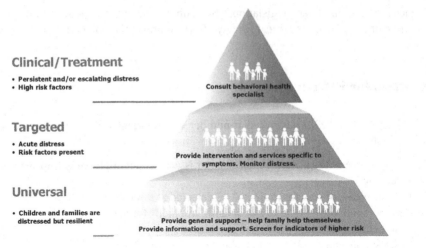

Fig. 12.1 The pediatric psychosocial preventative health model. (PPPHM; Kazak 2006)

Pai et al, 2008), they demonstrated that the PAT predicted psychosocial resource utilization and its cutoff scores correlated with standard measures of parent acute stress, child behavior problems, and family conflict.

For children with type 1 diabetes, our group developed and validated a 9-item interview to assess risk for poor glycemic control in newly-diagnosed type 1 diabetes patients, the Risk Index for Poor Glycemic Control (RI-PGC; Schwartz et al. 2013a). The measure was shown to have good sensitivity and specificity for poor glycemic control (A1c 9.5%), and was also able to identify patients at risk for DKA. Most importantly, it was designed for easy use and scoring by physicians and other medical providers. The nine items are scored as a simple sum which translates directly into an estimation of the absolute increase in risk associated with that score (Table 12.1).

Table 12.1. Use of the Risk Index for Poor Glycemic Control (RI-PGC) to estimate absolute increase in risk for poor glycemic control (HbA1c 9.5%), emergency room (ER) visits, and diabetic ketoacidosis (DKA). Predicted values are approximations accurate to within 10%. All values are rounded to the nearest multiple of five for ease of use. (From Schwartz et al. 2013a)

RI-PGC score	Poor glycemic control (%)	ER visits (%)	DKA (%)
0	+0	+0	+0
1	+10	+5	+5
2	+20	+15	+20
3	+35	+25	+20
4	+40	+30	+30
5	>+40	>+30	+40

A more extensive interview that provides broader coverage of psychosocial risk factors has also been developed. The Psychosocial Risk Screening Measure (PRiSM) is a 36-item semi-structured interview assessing risk in five domains known to be important risk factors for poor diabetes control (Schwartz et al. 2010): sociodemographic factors such as race/ethnicity and SES; child problems (e.g., behavior or mood problems); family conflict; caregiver problems (e.g., depression); and anticipated diabetes-related problems (e.g., anticipated conflict over diabetes management). These different domains have been organized into a "simple model" of risk for nonadherence (Fig. 12.2) that was used to guide development of the PRiSM screening tools (for a detailed description of the initial development of the screening tool, see Schwartz, Axelrad et al. 2011). The model assumes that the critical "actor" is the child/parent *team*, whose management abilities directly affect adherence, although they are also influenced by environmental factors and the healthcare team.

The PRiSM has been field-tested for feasibility and acceptability (Schwartz, Cline et al. 2011) and is currently being validated. A comprehensive training manual (and a supervisor's guide) that provides detailed instructions for using the RI-PGC and the PRiSM has been peer-reviewed (Schwartz et al. 2014) and is available for free download from MedEd Portal at www.mededportal.org/publication/9643. Moreover, we are also now developing modules for use with other pediatric populations, beginning with children with cancer.

Can problems be reliably identified after diagnosis? In established patients, there are many evidence-based assessment tools for nonadherence that have been validated in pediatric patients (see Quittner et al. 2008 for review). Typically these are questionnaires that are completed by the patient (if old enough) and/or the parent.

Psychosocial screening tools can also be used to detect risk for nonadherence when there is a well documented relationship between the risk factor and the outcome. For example, Hilliard et al. (2011) used brief, validated measures of depression (Children's Depression Inventory) and anxiety (the state scale of the State-Trait Anxiety Inventory for Children) to predict adherence (blood glucose monitoring frequency) and glycemic control (HbA1c) in youth age 13–18 with type 1 diabetes

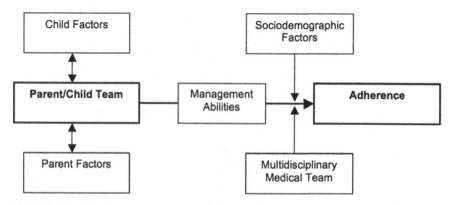

Fig. 12.2 The "Simple Model" of risk for nonadherence. (Schwartz et al. 2010)

1 year later. Symptoms of depression predicted reduced blood glucose monitoring, and anxiety predicted poorer glycemic control, possibly due to concurrent associations with stress.

Healthcare providers can also assess for nonadherence more informally. While informal assessment is more prone to individual biases and lack of sensitivity to uncovering problems, it is often the only option available to clinicians in busy routine practice. Moreover, simply asking patients about current problems can be valuable in its own right, as it has been shown to relate to an improved therapeutic relationship. Healthcare providers can start by acknowledging that most patients struggle with managing aspects of the medical regimen, and then ask what parts of the regimen are difficult for the patient. Assessing specific behaviors (e.g., frequency of blood glucose checks) is critical. Providers can also ask more general questions about the burden of illness management. Peyrot and Rubin (2007) suggest asking patients:

• Do you feel overwhelmed or burned out by the demands of illness management?
• Do you get the support you need from your family for illness management?

A downside of informal questioning is that it can be difficult to interpret findings and compare findings across patients, and important areas might be missed.

Is screening feasible and acceptable to patients and their families? Feasibility of screening is threatened by its potential burden on patients/families, healthcare providers, and the system of routine care. As noted earlier, screening services are often not reimbursable, and they can be quite resource-intensive in terms of administration, scoring, and interpretation. To address these problems in screening newly diagnosed cancer patients, Kazak et al. (2011) arranged for nursing staff to administer the measure to patients, who completed it as a questionnaire. They reported an 88 % completion and return rate, and 98 % of cases were scored, reviewed, and shared with the treatment team within a couple of days. They also reported a high degree of buy-in from nursing leadership and staff.

We took a different approach to screening newly diagnosed type 1 diabetes patients. For clinical reasons, we believed it was important to use a face-to-face interview approach rather than a questionnaire. Conducting interviews allowed us to provide appropriate support to families throughout the assessment process; a secondary goal was to put a "face" on psychology to reduce potential stigma (Schwartz, Axelrad et al. 2011). To staff this service, we incorporated the screening into our training program for pediatric psychology pre-doctoral interns and fellows. In an initial feasibility study (Schwartz, Cline et al. 2011), we were able to screen 75 % of patients, with an almost 97 % participation rate (121 out of 125 families approached). A subset of families ($n=30$) completed satisfaction ratings, with a satisfaction score of 90 %, reflecting an average rating of 4.5 out of 5 (Very Good to Excellent). No one rated the service "fair" or "poor."

Is there effective intervention for identified problems? As discussed in Chap. 4, there are a multitude of effective, evidence-based approaches to treating nonadherence in pediatric patients that also have beneficial effects on children's health. They do tend to be resource intensive, however, typically requiring implementation by a well-trained behavioral health specialist (although there are exceptions; Anderson et al. 1999). As a result, most of the proven interventions have been focused on patients with clinically significant needs. Interventions at different levels of risk are clearly needed.

There are also effective interventions for related psychosocial concerns such as depression. For example, in a meta-analysis of intervention studies targeting internalizing problems (e.g., depression, anxiety), externalizing behavior problems, coping skills, and health beliefs in children with cancer, cystic fibrosis, sickle cell disease, and type 1 diabetes, Beale (2006) found a mean effect size of $d=0.71$ across illness types, which he noted translates into improvement for 80% of participants.

Concerns About Screening

As noted by many authors, universal screening raises a number of important ethical issues. First is the issue of informed consent. We believe it is very important for families to understand *why* a screening is being conducted, and to provide informed consent (and assent for minor children) for the procedure. To this end we have developed very stringent consent procedures around our diabetes screening process, as detailed in the training manual (Schwartz et al. 2013).

Second, many providers express concern about asking about psychosocial risk factors at or near the time of disease diagnosis, which is usually a fraught and stressful time for most patients and their families. This is an understandable concern, though we believe it is probably unfounded in most cases. In our experience screening newly diagnosed children with type 1 diabetes (over 600 patients to date), very few families have had any sort of complaint; instead, the vast majority have commented on how helpful it was to have someone to talk to about these concerns. It did help that our interviewers were all well trained in psychological interviewing and in helping families manage stress.

Third is the issue of false positive and false negatives. *False positives* are often a concern in medicine, as a false positive test can result in unnecessary procedures, treatments, and expenses, potentially placing a substantial extra burden on patients and their families. In addition, false positives can be stressful and frightening, as when a person is told he has a condition with significant long-term implications. These are important considerations. However, we would argue that the problem of false positives is small if not negligible in the realm of adherence. The usual outcome of a positive result is a conversation between the clinician and the patient and parent, in which it can be determined whether the family is interested (and sees a need) for further evaluation and/or treatment—hardly a bad thing.

Given the above considerations, we suggest that screening for nonadherence err on the side of over-sensitivity—i.e., to set parameters such that one is more likely to have a false positive than a false negative. Indeed, others have suggested considering anything less than 100% reported adherence as suggestive of a possible adherence problem, given that self-report tends to inflate rates of adherence (Marhefka et al. 2006; Steele and Grauer 2003).

However, *false negatives* can also be of some concern, as they can give rise to a false sense of security, and because a condition may therefore go untreated. Again, though, this problem seems relatively minimal with regards to nonadherence. After all, if a child has poor illness control without obvious nonadherent behaviors or psychosocial comorbidities, the illness can still be treated from a medical perspective. For example, in surveillance screenings we have been conducting with established type 1 diabetes patients, we have found the following pattern in some patients: high HbA1c, parent- and/or self-report of feeling overwhelmed by diabetes, no other concerns (e.g., no nonadherence, no depression or behavior problems, etc), and no interest in psychological follow-up. In these cases, we have been recommending further consultation with the treating endocrinologist around simplifying the medical regimen, and so far anecdotal evidence suggests that this has been helpful, although more data are needed to know whether this pattern is in fact "real."

Tips to Assessing for Nonadherence

Providers may find the following "tips" and suggestions useful in helping them assess for nonadherence in their pediatric patients. Asking questions can have beneficial effects on the provider-patient relationship, but it should be noted that it cannot take the place of standardized assessment in cases where it is indicated. An effective approach might be to routinely ask some subset of these questions, to be followed up with a validated measure if some concern comes to light.

1. Prior to meeting the patient, look for biomarkers (e.g., high HbA1c) without alternate explanation
   a. But do not assume that the patient is nonadherent even if it seems obvious
   b. Do not confront the patient, or use scare tactics
2. Take a minute to develop rapport—you cannot learn anything if the family distrusts you
3. Meet with the child—give him or her the choice of meeting with you alone or with the parent present. Even children as young as 5 can benefit from some direct interaction with the provider.
4. Ask the child:
   a. What are the most difficult parts of living with/taking care of ___?
   b. How would ___ have to change for you to feel/do better?
   c. What steps could you take to improve the problem?
   d. What changes are you willing to make?
   e. How can we (therapist, parent) help you take these steps/make these changes?
5. With older children, ask about:
   a. Family support and conflict—e.g.,
      i. Do you feel that you get enough support from your family around ___?
      ii. Do you and your parents ever fight over managing ___?
   b. Burnout—"Do you ever feel tired or just burned out over managing ___?

(See Peyrot and Rubin 2007; Schwartz, Axelrad et al. 2011; Wysocki 1997.)

Summary and Conclusions

In this chapter we have reviewed the evidence supporting the value of screening for nonadherence and contributory psychosocial risk factors. However, screening is not without its costs. It can be resource intensive, and challenging for clinicians practicing outside of major medical centers to implement. However, validated screening tools such as the PAT and the RI-PGC, which were designed for easy use in routine practice, may help extend the reach and feasibility of screening.

Nonetheless, moving forward into the new era of healthcare, it will be critically important to demonstrate that risk screening can indeed *prevent* costly complications, and show its cost effectiveness. For example, it has been shown that risk screening at diabetes diagnosis can predict subsequent emergency room visits over the next 9 months (Schwartz, Cline et al. 2011). Specifically, children from single-parent households who also had behavior problems were much more likely to end up back in the ER for a diabetes-related concern. As there are well-established and very effective interventions for child behavior problems (Axelrad et al. 2009; Child and Adolescent Mental Health Division Evidence Based Services Committee 2007; Eyberg et al. 2008), preventive interventions focused on these high-risk children have the potential to substantially reduce the incidence of expensive ER visits.

At the same time, we also need interventions developed for children who are at-risk but do not have (as of yet) clinically significant concerns, as well as more universal interventions focused on preventing the emergence of risk factors such as normative family conflict. Interventions aimed at these lower acuity patients, if implemented widely enough, could have broad effects on the health of the population of children with chronic disease. In the next chapter, we present a model for implementing a tiered, multi-modal intervention framework for providing intervention services at *all* levels of risk—Universal, Targeted, and Clinical—as delineated in Kazak's (2006) PPPHM.

References

Anderson B, Brackett J, Ho J, Laffel LM. An office-based intervention to maintain parent-adolescent teamwork in diabetes management. Impact on parent involvement, family conflict, and subsequent glycemic control. Diabetes Care. 1999;22:713–21.

Anderson BJ, Vangsness L, Connell A, Butler D, Goebel-Fabbri A, Laffel LMB. Family conflict, adherence, and glycaemic control in youth with short duration type 1 diabetes. Diab Med. 2002;19:635–42.

Axelrad M, Garland B, Love K. Brief behavioral intervention for young children with disruptive behaviors. J Clin Psychol Med Settings. 2009;16:263–9.

Beale IL. Scholarly literature review: efficacy of psychological interventions for pediatric chronic illnesses. J Pediatr Psychol. 2006;31:437–51.

Cameron FJ, Northam EA, Ambler G, Daneman D. Routine psychological screening in youth with type 1 diabetes and their parents: a notion whose time has come? Diabetes Care. 2007;30:2716–24.

Child and Adolescent Mental Health Division Evidence Based Services Committee. 2007 Biennial Report: effective psychosocial interventions for youth with behavioral and emotional needs. 2007.

Cline VD, Schwartz DD, Axelrad ME, Anderson BJ. A pilot study of acute stress symptoms in parents and youth following diagnosis of type 1 diabetes. Journal of Clinical Psychology in Medical Settings 2011; 18: 16–22.

De Civita M, Dobkin PL. Pediatric adherence as a multidimensional and dynamic construct, involving a triadic partnership. J Ped Psychol. 2004;29:157–69.

Eyberg SM, Nelson MM, Boggs SR. Evidence-based psychosocial treatment for children and adolescents with disruptive behavior. J Clin Child Adol Psychol. 2008;37:215–37.

Gates TJ. Screening for cancer: evaluating the evidence. Am Fam Physician 2001; 63(3): 513–523.

Grey M, Cameron M, Lipman TH, Thurber FW. Psychosocial status of children with diabetes in the first 2 years after diagnosis. Diabetes Care. 1995;18:1330–6.

Hilliard ME, Herzer M, Dolan LM, Hood KK. Psychological screening in adolescents with type 1 diabetes predicts outcomes one year later. Diab Res Clin Pract. 2011;94:39–44.

Hood KK, Huestis S, Maher A, Butler D, Volkening L, Laffel LM. Depressive symptoms in children and adolescents with type 1 diabetes: association with diabetes-specific characteristics. Diabetes Care. 2006;29:1389–91.

Kazak AE. Pediatric psychosocial preventative health model (PPPHM): research, practice and collaboration in pediatric family systems medicine. Fam Syst Health. 2006;24:381–95.

Kazak AE, Prusak A, McSherry M, et al. The psychosocial assessment tool (PAT): development of a brief screening instrument for identifying high risk families in pediatric oncology. Fam Syst Health. 2001;19:303–17.

Kazak AE, Cant MC, Jensen MM, et al. Identifying psychosocial risk indicative of subsequent resource utilization in families of newly diagnosed pediatric oncology patients. J Clin Oncol. 2003; 21:3220–25; J Pediatr Psychol. 2008;33(1):50–62.

Kazak AE, Barakat LP, Ditaranto S, et al. Screening for psychosocial risk at cancer diagnosis: the Psychosocial Assessment Tool (PAT). J Pediatr Hematol Oncol. 2011;33:289–94.

Kocher R, Emanuel EJ, DeParle NAM. The Affordable Care Act and the future of clinical medicine: the opportunities and challenges. Annals Intern Med. 2010;153:536–9.

Koh HK, Sebelius KG. Promoting prevention through the affordable care act. N Engl J Med. 2010;363:1296–9.

Kovacs M, Goldston D, Obrosky S, Iyengar S. Prevalence and predictors of pervasive non-compliance with medical treatment among youths with insulin-dependent diabetes mellitus. J Am Acad Child Adol Psychiatry. 1992;31:1112–9.

Marhefka SL, Tepper VJ, Brown JL, Farley JJ. Caregiver psychosocial characteristics and children's adherence to antiretroviral therapy. AIDS Patient Care STDS. 2006;20:429–37.

Modi AC, Guilfoyle SM, Rausch JR. Preliminary feasibility, acceptability, and efficacy of an innovative adherence intervention for children with newly diagnosed epilepsy. Journal of Pediatric Psychology. 2013:38, 605–616.

Morrison AS. Screening in chronic disease. 2nd ed. New York: Oxford University Press; 1992.

Morrison A. Screening. In: Rothman K, Greenland S, Editors. Modern epidemiology. 2nd ed. Philadelphia: Lippincott-Raven; 1998. pp. 499–518.

Pai AL, Patiño-Fernández AM, McSherry M, et al. The Psychosocial Assessment Tool (PAT2.0): Psychometric properties of a screener for psychosocial distress in families of children newly diagnosed with cancer. J Pediatr Psychol. 2008;33:50–62.

Peyrot M, Rubin RR. Behavioral and psychosocial interventions in diabetes a conceptual review. Diabetes Care. 2007;30:2433–40.

Phillips LA, Leventhal EA, Leventhal H. Factors associated with the accuracy of physicians' predictions of patient adherence. Patient Educ Couns 2011;85:461–7.

Quittner AL, Modi AC, Lemanek KL, Ievers-Landis CE, Rapoff MA. Evidence-based assessment of adherence to medical treatments in pediatric psychology. J Pediatr Psychol 2008;33:916–36.

Sabate E. Adherence to long-term therapies: evidence for action. Geneva: World Health Organization; 2003.

Schwartz DD, Cline VD, Hansen J, Axelrad ME, Anderson BJ. Early risk factors for nonadherence in pediatric type 1 diabetes: a review of the recent literature. Curr Diabetes Rev. 2010;6:167–83.

Schwartz DD, Axelrad ME, Cline VD, Anderson BJ. A model psychosocial screening program for children and youth with newly diagnosed type 1 diabetes: implications for psychologists across contexts of care. Prof Psychol: Res Prac. 2011;42:324–30.

Schwartz DD, Cline VD, Axelrad ME, Anderson BJ. Feasibility, acceptability, and predictive validity of a psychosocial screening program for children and youth newly diagnosed with type 1 diabetes. Diabetes Care. 2011;34:326–31.

Schwartz D, Axelrad M, Anderson B. Psychosocial risk screening of children newly diagnosed with type 1 diabetes: a training toolkit for healthcare professionals. MedEdPORTAL; 2013. www.mededportal.org/publication/9643.

Schwartz, DD, Axelrad ME, Anderson BJ. A psychosocial risk index for poor glycemic control in children and adolescents with Type 1 diabetes. Pediatr Diabetes 2014; 15: 190–197.

Stark L. Introduction to the special issue on adherence in pediatric medical conditions. J Pediatr Psychol. 2013;38:589–94.

Steele RG, Grauer D. Adherence to antiretroviral therapy for pediatric HIV infection: review of the literature and recommendations for research. *Clin Child Fam Psychol Rev.* 2003;6: 17–30.

US Preventive Services Task Force. Screening and treatment for major depressive disorder in children and adolescents: US Preventive Services Task Force recommendation statement. Pediatrics. 2009;123:1223–28.

Wolfsdorf J, Craig ME, Daneman D, Dunger D, Edge J, Lee W, Rosenbloom A, Sperling M, Hanas R. Diabetic ketoacidosis in children and adolescents with diabetes. Pediatr Diabetes. 2009;10:118–33.

Writing Team for the Diabetes Control and Complications Trial/Epidemiology of Diabetes Interventions and Complications Research Group. Sustained effect of intensive treatment of type 1 diabetes mellitus on development and progression of diabetic nephropathy: the epidemiology of diabetes interventions and complications (EDIC) study. JAMA 2003;290:2159–67.

Wysocki T. The ten keys to helping your child grow up with diabetes. Alexandria: American Diabetes Association; 1997.

Chapter 13
A Comprehensive Behavioral Health System for Identifying and Treating Nonadherence

Abstract In this chapter we describe an innovative system designed to promote adherence, prevent nonadherence, and provide interventions for nonadherence based on level and type of risk. While there are many discrete interventions focused on adherence being implemented at institutions across the country, they tend to be highly focused in terms of method and target population. The model sketched out here provides a different approach, focused on improving the overall system in which treatment takes place, rather than placing the entire burden of treatment adherence on the patient (or patient and parent) alone. The system utilizes a web-based hub and incorporates universal screening for risk for nonadherence at disease diagnosis; triage to targeted interventions; and ongoing surveillance for newly emerging adherence problems or psychosocial concerns. In the model, interventions are based on level and type of assessed risk or need. At the Universal level (low risk patients), we provide examples of preventive educational materials and tools that can be given to patients and parents. At the Targeted (moderate risk) level, we delineate using outreach supports as efficient ways to mitigate risk by keeping at-risk patients and families connected to, and helping them navigate, the healthcare system. For children assessed to be at the Clinical (highest risk) level, we provide guidelines for referral for individualized intervention. We end the chapter with a summary of the key factors and guiding principles for developing an effective system-based approach to adherence.

Overview of the Comprehensive Model

If we are to be successful in helping children and their families live with and manage a chronic illness and stay healthy physically and mentally, risk factors for nonadherence in multiple areas will need to be addressed in a systematic fashion (Sabate 2003). Specifically, a comprehensive program will need to address all of the risk domains indicated in the "simple model" presented in the last chapter: patient factors (e.g., health beliefs, depression); parent and family factors (e.g., parent mental health); parent/child teamwork (communication, conflict); healthcare provider behaviors that influence adherence (e.g., communication style); and socioeconomic factors that affect families' ability to obtain care and navigate the healthcare system.

© Springer International Publishing Switzerland 2015

D. D. Schwartz, M. E. Axelrad, *Healthcare Partnerships for Pediatric Adherence,*
SpringerBriefs in Public Health, DOI 10.1007/978-3-319-13668-4_13

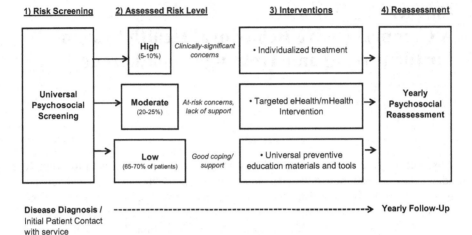

Fig. 13.1 The comprehensive model of pediatric adherence promotion, showing patient flow from risk assessment through triage and intervention, to yearly reassessment

To be successful, the system would need mechanisms for (1) screening/assessment of risk and current problems; (2) triage to different interventions based on the overall level of assessed risk (low, moderate, or high) and on the type of risk (sociodemographic; problems with child, caregiver, or family functioning; disease-specific concerns); and (3) reassessment on a periodic basis. Moreover, these different components would need to be integrated into a cohesive whole. Figure 13.1 shows the process flow, from entry into the system to yearly re-evaluation. Each component of this process is described below.

Universal Psychosocial Screening at Diagnosis The first part of the process—and the entry point into the system—is through an initial psychosocial screening (Chap. 12). Ideally this would occur at disease diagnosis, although it might occur at the first new patient visit; when the system is first rolled out, established patients would also need an initial screening. Screening could be completed by interview or via a standardized questionnaire. We recommend using a screening tool that could be used to categorize level of risk (or need for established patients). Measures designed to do this include the RI-PGC for children and youth with type 1 diabetes (Schwartz et al. 2014) and the PAT for children/youth with cancer (Kazak et al. 2011).

Assessed Risk Triage is based on assessed risk level. Following Kazak's PPPHM (Kazak 2006), the model defines three risk levels or categories of need, as shown in Table 13.1. Assessed risk level then determines the type and intensity of intervention. Important risk factors include:

- Low SES
- Single-parent family
- Caregiver unemployment

Table 13.1 The risk categorization model and indications for intervention

Risk level	Characterization	Indication for intervention
High risk (Clinical)	Clinically significant concerns with child or family functioning	Individualized treatment
Moderate risk	Risk factors for problematic adjustment or adherence Limited resources	Preventive low-level interventions designed to minimize risk and keep the child and family connected to the healthcare system
Low risk	Good coping, good support, adequate resources	Universal educational resources and illness management tools

- Child behavioral or psychological concerns
- Parent mental health problems
- Family conflict (including marital conflict)
- A current history of nonadherence (established patients)

As a rough rule of thumb, having two risk factors (or one risk factor plus poor illness control) would place a patient in the *moderate risk category*, and three or more risk factors would place a child in the *high risk category* (Schwartz et al. 2014). However, problem severity and parent distress/desire for intervention should also be taken into account when making this determination. For example, a child with significant behavior problems but no other concerns would likely still warrant clinical intervention.

Interventions Interventions should be offered based on assessed level of risk/need to ensure efficient allocation of resources and to cover the range of needs, from universal education to clinical intervention. Below we give an overview of the type of intervention indicated at each level, according to current evidence-based practice in behavioral health. The actual interventions are described in greater detail in the sections that follow.

Importantly, patients at higher levels of assessed need should also have access to interventions at lower levels. Thus, moderate risk patients would have access to the educational materials and management tools as well as to targeted interventions, and high risk patients would have access to all of the different intervention components.

- *High risk.* Patients assessed to have clinically-significant concerns should be seen by or referred to a pediatric psychologist or other specialist in behavioral or mental health, for individually tailored intervention. High acuity patients (e.g., with suicidal ideation) would probably need to be seen outside of the system being presented here.
- *Moderate risk.* Moderate risk patients are characterized either by a single child or family-related risk factor (e.g., family conflict), or by one or more resource limitations. The primary goals for these patients should be to minimize risk,

prevent complications, and help keep the family tied in to the system. Thus, appropriate supports at this level would be targeted interventions focused on the specific area of risk identified (e.g., child behavior problem), help obtaining resources (e.g., from a social worker), and/or support for navigating the healthcare system (via a patient navigator or Care Ambassador (see below), depending on specific needs.

- *Low risk* patients have adequate coping and supports. The indicated intervention at this level would be universal educational materials, and access to illness management tools that could make living with and managing their disease easier.

Yearly Psychosocial Reassessment For many patients, problems with adherence do not emerge until they have lived with the illness for a while. Some children and youth may experience management burnout (Polonsky 1996). Others may pass through the developmental transition into adolescence, a time during which illness management and control is known to be especially challenging, or may encounter other stressors that complicate management. As a result, continued monitoring of patients' adherence and psychosocial functioning is critical.

A Web-Based System for Evidence-Based Intervention at All Levels of Risk/need

Designing and implementing this sort of comprehensive system is by no means easy. Significant resources need to be available to address each component, and the model needs to be sustainable over time. To accomplish this, we believe use of an internet-based hub could make implementation feasible. A web-based hub could house the educational materials and tools, utilize software for screening, provide a platform for eHealth and mHealth interventions, and link patients to clinical staff, care navigators, and the larger patient community (Fig. 11).

Web-based interventions have be shown to be effective in promoting health and reducing nonadherence across a wide-range of illnesses. They also have substantial ability for improving the reach, accessibility, effectiveness, and cost-effectiveness of interventions (Bennett and Glasgow 2009; Murray 2012). Internet–based programs have the potential to disseminate effective interventions to very large groups of people, making them an ideal format for large-scale efforts at health promotion. Their large reach helps ensure that even small changes across a population can have a substantial impact on public health (Murray 2012).

Internet and mobile technologies have a high level of uptake among children, teens, and young adults, having been integrated into their lives in an unprecedented fashion. As such, these technologies provide a natural way to monitor patients' health and well-being, provide them with reminders and other contact, and keep them connected to their healthcare on weekly or even daily basis, with a relatively low "footprint" and minimal intrusiveness into their daily lives. eHealth and

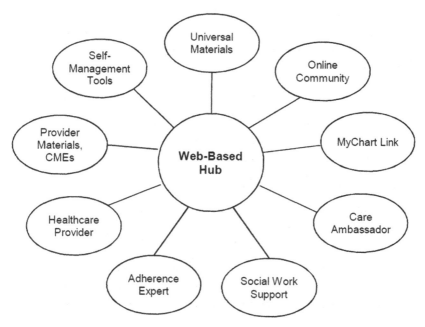

Fig. 13.2 A web-based hub linking patients to services at different levels

mHealth interventions also have the potential to be more acceptable to patients who would be reluctant to go see a psychologist or psychiatrist, thereby increasing the reach of effective services to patients who might otherwise "fall through the cracks."

In the next section we describe how a web-based hub could be used to link and integrate the different components of a multi-level, multimodal system for promoting adherence. We sketch out a system with two access points: a public portal, freely open and available to the public; and a patient portal, accessible only to patients being treated at a specific institution (Fig. 13.2).

Universal Preventive Services

The Public Portal

Universal educational resources and tools could be provided for patients and the public at large as a primary prevention strategy to help promote treatment adherence. To be most effective, materials should be developed specifically for different age groups (children, teens, and parents), and in some cases also for specific-diseases.

Important educational resources to consider for inclusion in the public portal include:

- Basic information on medical treatments for specific (targeted) medical populations, including best practice treatment guidelines abstracted from the current literature and written in a patient-friendly format
- Disease-specific information on high risk behaviors—e.g., insulin omission in diabetes
- Adherence "tips" and informational pages on topics such as problem-solving, stress management, and managing family conflict
- Patient essays and videos presenting personal stories about challenges and successes in managing different chronic illnesses
- Links to local, regional, and national resources

Important web-based tools to help with illness management include:

- Customizable medication reminders linked to the patient's phone
- Customizable appointment reminders
- An interactive problem-solver program to help patients develop possible solutions to common adherence problems and barriers
- A nonadherence risk assessment tool (e.g., the RI-PGC; Schwartz et al. 2014, in which the user answers a few questions and receives a computer-generated risk estimate for possible nonadherence with linked suggestions for seeking further care.

The website could also be used to house professionally monitored discussion forum(s), to provide access to a patient community. It would be important for these forums to have lower age limits (e.g., 12 and older), to be disease-specific, and to be carefully monitored for potentially harmful information (e.g., diabetic teens sharing the information that omitting insulin can be an effective way to control weight).

The Patient Portal

In addition to the universal materials and tools suggested above, patients in participating clinics could also be given access to tools and supports linked to their medical chart and to the hospital/clinic where they receive their treatment. Of course, security concerns in designing this system would be paramount, to ensure that only the patient (and his/her legal guardians) would have access to the information. The following elements would be important to include:

1. Patient-specific health information
   - A link to the patient's medical chart
   - A downloadable summary of the patient's current treatment regimen (prepared by his/her healthcare provider), formatted to be maximally useful and easy to read
2. Tools linking the patient to different parts of the healthcare system
   - An automatic appointment reminder tool linked to the hospital/clinic system
   - Assistance with medication refills, linked to the patient's pharmacy

3. Adherence-related supportsThese could be provided by an "expert" in adherence. The expert could be a psychologist, a supervised predoctoral resident or postdoctoral fellow in psychology, or a licensed Masters-level counselor with training in behavioral health. Important services include:
   - A monitored email address for adherence-related questions
   - Ask the Expert—online help for adherence-related difficulties, provided through an instant messaging format at pre-specified times during the week
   - Ability to request an appointment with an adherence specialist
4. Access to a psychosocial screening tool for yearly reassessment
   Yearly face-to-face follow-up screening would probably not be feasible for large clinics and hospitals, if done on a universal scale (although it would work just fine in a small clinic setting). To accomplish follow-up screenings, a computerized screening tool could be built into the integrated system and access over the hub. Patients could receive yearly reminders to log in and complete the screen; in addition, they could access the tool any time they want to complete a self-assessment. The tool could operate as a nomogram, using pre-programmed algorithms to calculate risk and provide immediate feedback to the user in a patient-friendly format, with a recommendation for follow-up care as indicated based on level and type of risk.

Specific risk factors could also be linked to appropriate materials and tools also located on the hub. For example:

- A parent reporting moderate conflict over illness management could be directed to educational materials on reducing/managing conflict
- A parent indicating socioeconomic risk and lack of insurance could be linked directly to social work support
- A parent reporting multiple risk factors could be given a recommendation for psychology follow-up, including a link to request a follow-up appointment

To make the system truly integrated into clinical practice, screening results could also be emailed to the treating provider (and/or to the adherence expert if one is on staff), who could review the information, place it in the patients electronic medical record, and contact the patient (if an adult) or the parent via email if any problems are indicated.

Mobile App

Creation of a mobile phone app linked directly into the website would greatly increase the system's reach.

Targeted Services

Another benefit of the website is that it could provide the infrastructure for actually providing targeted eHealth interventions to patients assessed to be at risk for problems with adherence, or who are currently experiencing mild to moderate problems limited (or mostly limited) to adherence. Interventions would be low intensity, and offered with the understanding that they would not take the place of working with an actual provider.

Patients and families identified as appropriate for web-based services could be given information about the program at a clinic visit by their healthcare provider or during an in-clinic consultation by the adherence expert, and encouraged to sign up for the intervention through the Patient Portal. (Patients with clinically-significant mental health concerns should be triaged to individualized treatment with a psychologist or other mental health provider.)

Important features of effective eHealth interventions include:

- *Tailoring interventions* to individual patients based on the specific risk factors identified through the screening. For example, parents who report behavior problems in their school-age children might be directed to educational modules on parent management skills; families in which there is a high level of parent-child conflict might be guided to educational modules on communication skills and conflict resolution; and teens who report feeling stressed and burned out might be guided to modules on stress management.
- *Goal-setting, readiness for change, and action plan development tools*. For example, patients receiving a targeted intervention could first be guided to a goal-setting program, where they would be able to define their own goals for health or behavior change, have the opportunity to explore their readiness for change, and consider factors that might help or hinder them from making this change. These factors in turn could be incorporated into the action plan the patient develops with the guidance of the program.
- *Problem solving*. If patients run into difficulty with setting or reaching goals, they could have access to a module that would walk them through a series of problem-solving steps to help try to figure out the problem and devise (or revise) a plan for moving forward toward their goal.
- *Expert advice*. An important aspect of providing eHealth interventions is that there would be an actual person, with expertise in adherence, to provide guidance to the family as they use the online tool. This could be done through an "Ask the Expert" service done over email or via online help through instant messaging at pre-specified times. The focus would have to be specifically on adherence, not questions about the medical regimen, which would be routed to the healthcare provider.
- *Check-ins*. If resources allow, patients and parents might also be given the opportunity to request "check-ins" from the adherence expert to see how they are doing with the program, and more generally with their adaption to living with a chronic illness. The purpose would be to help patients feel connected and personally cared for (to give a human voice to the intervention). Patients could define a time frame (daily, every few days, weekly, never, etc) and a modality (email, text message, chat) in which they prefer to be contacted.
- *Questions*. It would also be important to have a mechanism for patients and parents to have adherence-related questions answered in a timely fashion. This

could be done by providing contact information for a Care Ambassador (see below), who could route questions to the appropriate person (medical questions to their healthcare provider, adherence questions to an adherence expert, insurance and billing questions to appropriate staff, etc). Alternately, direct email links to appropriate clinical and office staff could be provided.

Keeping Patients Connected

An important although understudied area related to adherence has to do with patients and families "losing touch" with the clinic and their healthcare providers. This is especially true among minority patients (Schwartz et al. 2010). The integrated system could provide a cost-effective means to keep patients connected. Ways to accomplish this include generating reminders (e.g., for appointments) and sending check-in messages (e.g., via text message) to see how patients are doing.

Patients could also be provided with the services of a *Care Ambassador* (Laffel et al. 1998). Care Ambassadors provide outreach to patients and families to help them stay connected to the medical clinic and navigate the healthcare system. The intervention is designed to help patients and their families receive ambulatory diabetes care as prescribed by the patient's usual diabetes health care team. Care Ambassadors provide no prescriptive advice. Rather, they encourage patients and their families to seek medical advice from their health care team in a timely manner. In this respect, they are comparable to office personnel usually found in a medical setting. Typical duties include: assisting families with appointment scheduling and confirmation; helping families with questions concerning billing or insurance by directing them to the appropriate personnel; monitoring clinic attendance, and providing telephone or written outreach to families after missed or canceled appointments.

Care Ambassadors have the ability to follow a caseload of approximately 40–50 families. The intervention could be targeted to patients and families found to be at highest risk for missing clinic appointments and being lost to follow-up. Outreach interventions of this sort may be especially important for impoverished, single-parent, and minority families, for whom much of the risk for nonadherence comes from feeling disenfranchised and disconnected from the healthcare system.

The Care Ambassador intervention has solid empirical support. Compared to standard care, children with Care Ambassador support services attended over a third more clinic appointments; were half as likely to have severe hyperglycemia; and had 25% fewer total hypoglycemic events, 60% fewer severe hypoglycemic events, and 40% fewer hospitalizations and emergency department visits in a large 2-year prospective RCT (Laffel et al. 1998; Svoren et al. 2003).

Training for Healthcare Professionals

Another critical aspect of promoting adherence is changing healthcare provider behavior. Research indicates that some providers still view nonadherence through the lens of compliance (especially with minority patients), and many communicate poorly with patients, with negative effects on adherence. To address this an integrated website could also house materials for providers, including:

- CME modules on topics such as: Understanding Adherence; Improving Patient Adherence; Fostering Family Teamwork; and Improving Communication with Your Patients.
- Patient education materials for healthcare providers to use with their patients on a range of adherence-related topics.

Summary of the Integrated Behavioral Health System

The comprehensive system outlined here is offered as a model for providing integrated care around adherence promotion in a way that is resource savvy and sustainable. Table 13.2 provides a summary of the key components and the domains they are intended to help address. More broadly, critical facets of the model are:

Its ability to make changes across multiple levels. Patients do not manage a chronic illness in a vacuum. Families, healthcare providers, and the healthcare system all play substantial roles in helping foster a patient's treatment adherence. Fostering changes at all of these levels simultaneously has the potential to affect adherence in ways that single-target interventions may not be able to accomplish.

Its ability to provide low intensity services to at-risk patients. Few interventions focus on the middle of the risk pyramid (Fig. 8), the at-risk patients who are not (yet) experiencing clinically-significant concerns. Preventing complications in this large group of children is a critical but overlooked priority.

Its focus on prevention. Interventions focused on preventing or reducing acute life-threatening complications of nonadherence can have a greater impact on children's health than attempts to intervene after problems have occurred. Medical crises and related hospitalizations account for the lion's share of morbidity, mortality, and cost in patients with chronic illness. In addition, the preventive approach taken here helps "set the stage" for better long-term illness control, as adherence behaviors are known to be established in the first years following diagnosis, and good adherence early on can have a protective effect against later complications.

Its reach. The Catch-22 of adherence promotion is that the patients and families most in need of support often do not seek out or receive effective interventions. By using up-to-date technologies (internet, mobile apps) that have a high acceptability and uptake among pediatric populations, and linking this system to personal care, the methodology has the potential to reach many patients who otherwise might have "fallen through the cracks."

Its use of personal contact. Using a web-based system risks making intervention seem faceless and impersonal (and we doubt that this problem is solved by giving patients virtual "avatars," which is the approach used by some pharmaceutical companies on their websites). Linking the services with personal contact and personal-

Table 13.2 Summary of the suggested components for a behavioral health system. Web-based interventions could also be made accessible through a linked mobile phone app

Domain	Intervention	Format	Level
Knowledge	Educational patient materials	Website	Universal
Behavioral control	Management tools	Website	Universal
Social support/ social norms	Web-based social community (monitored chat rooms, bulletin boards, or forums)	Website	Universal
	Patient videos/stories		
Communication	Email, text messaging, chat	Website	Universal and Targeted (at-risk)
	Link to patient's EMR		
	Appointment reminders		
Connection with healthcare team	Support for navigating healthcare system	Website care ambassador	Targeted (at-risk)
	Personal appointment reminders		
Resources	Social work support	Social work	Targeted
Emotional support	Educational materials	Website	Universal
	Stress management modules		
	Patient videos/stories		
	User-defined check-ins via email, text, or chat	Adherence expert	Targeted (at-risk)
Family support	Educational modules on family teamwork	Website	Universal
	Family problem-solving tool		
	E-Health family intervention		Targeted (at-risk)
Significant child or family dysfunction	Behavioral/cognitive-behavioral therapy	Psychology/ behavioral health	Clinical
	Behavioral family therapy	Website	N/A
Provider behavior	Patient materials		
	CME modules		

ized care can help improve utilization of healthcare services and behavioral health interventions, thus further optimizing the system and its ability to have positive effects on a patient's life.

The behavioral health model proposed here represents an innovative attempt to address the widespread problem of suboptimal adherence proactively. By addressing multiple factors that support adherence more or less simultaneously, we believe this sort of integrated system has a better chance of effecting changes in overall adherence rates. A corollary of this approach is that takes as a basic assumption that illness management results from the efforts of multiple actors operating within multiple contexts, and that communication is a key to coordinating these efforts and fostering effective teamwork.

The initial development of this sort of integrated system is likely to be somewhat costly and resource-intensive, and maintaining it will also not be resource-free, especially if (as we recommend) it incorporates personnel such as Care Ambassadors and an adherence expert, and is kept up-to-date to reflect increasing knowledge and changes in the field. Demonstrating its cost effectiveness, perhaps primarily by reducing incidence of acute medical crises requiring hospitalization, will therefore be critical, as will demonstrating its clinical effectiveness through rigorous empirical investigations. Nonetheless, the hope is that this sort of model main gain traction in the new healthcare environment, in which there will be greater incentives to promote adherence and demonstrate positive health outcomes (Stark 2013).

References

Bennett GG, Glasgow RE. The delivery of public health interventions via the Internet: actualizing their potential. Ann Rev Public Health. 2009;30:273–92.

Kazak AE. Pediatric Psychosocial Preventative Health Model (PPPHM): research, practice and collaboration in pediatric family systems medicine. Families Syst Health. 2006;24:381–95.

Kazak AE, Barakat LP, Ditaranto S, et al. Screening for psychosocial risk at cancer diagnosis: the Psychosocial Assessment Tool (PAT). J Pediatr Hematol Oncol. 2011;33:289–94.

Laffel L, Brackett J, Ho J, Anderson BJ. Changing the process of diabetes care improves metabolic outcomes and reduces hospitalizations. Qual Manag Health Care. 1998;6:53–62.

Murray E. Web-based interventions for behavior change and self-management: potential, pitfalls, and progress. Medicine 2.0. 2012;1:e3.

Polonsky WH. Understanding and treating patients with diabetes burnout. Practical psychology for diabetes clinicians. Alexandria: American Diabetes Association; 1996. Pp. 183–92.

Sabate, E. Adherence to long-term therapies: evidence for action. Geneva: World Health Organization; 2003.

Schwartz DD, Cline VD, Hansen J, Axelrad ME, Anderson BJ. Early risk factors for nonadherence in pediatric type 1 diabetes: a review of the recent literature. Curr Diabetes Rev. 2010;6:167–83.

Schwartz, DD, Axelrad ME, Anderson BJ. A psychosocial risk index for poor glycemic control in children and adolescents with Type 1 diabetes. Pediatr Diabetes 2014; 15: 190–197

Stark L. Introduction to the special issue on adherence in pediatric medical conditions. J Pediatr Psychol. 2013;38:589–94.

Svoren B, Butler D, Levine B, Anderson B, Laffel L. Reducing acute adverse outcomes in youth with type 1 diabetes mellitus: a randomized controlled trial. Pediatrics. 2003;112:914–22.

Chapter 14
Pulling it All Together: Clinical Conclusions

Abstract In this final chapter, we summarize the ten most important take-home points from this volume on pediatric adherence in the context of the following main ideas. (1) Successful adherence depends on developing healthcare partnerships between patients, families, and providers, and that nonadherence often results from the breakdown of teamwork between any (or all) of the partners. (2) A focus on self-management instead of teamwork is likely to be self-defeating. Promoting patient independence too early risks a dangerous decline in illness management and control. In contrast, supporting patient autonomy (i.e., volitional behavior) can foster development without having to withdraw whatever assistance the youth may need. (3) Communication is the key to developing successful partnerships, which will usually be characterized by having shared goals and (ideally) a shared model of illness. We end this chapter—and the book—by highlighting the added value of partnerships for reducing the management burden chronic illness places on children.

Many articles and books have been dedicated to the investigation and improvement of patient adherence, yet suboptimal adherence remains a significant impediment to optimal levels of disease and illness control. This probably should not be surprising. There is often is little immediate benefit to expending all of the effort that goes into adherence. Moreover, it is not always clear that adherence even produces good results. For example, in a study of children with asthma, Kuehni and Frey (2002) found no differences in adherence between children with good and poor asthma control. Results of the meta-analysis by Graves et al. (2010) were reassuring in showing that improving adherence does *in general* result in better health outcomes, but even substantial improvements in public health do not always translate into improved quality of life for the individual.

Motivation for adherence may be improved by taking the onus off the individual patient and instead viewing adherence from the perspective of *family management*. Parents are often more motivated to ensure the long-term health of their children than their children are, and they are better able to take the long view. Seeing adherence as a family matter also takes some of the burden off the youth with a chronic illness—and that includes the burden of guilt and shame for poor disease control (often attributed by self and others to "doing a bad job"), as well as the substantial practical burdens of management. Wysocki (1997) suggested viewing problematic

© Springer International Publishing Switzerland 2015   175
D. D. Schwartz, M. E. Axelrad, *Healthcare Partnerships for Pediatric Adherence,*
SpringerBriefs in Public Health, DOI 10.1007/978-3-319-13668-4_14

adherence as reflecting the *breakdown of teamwork* around illness management, and we believe the value of this view cannot be overstated.

The evidence reviewed in this volume leads to some very clear and strong conclusions in this regard. First, neither children nor adolescents can manage an illness on their own. Chronic illnesses are complex, heavy burdens that require planning, organization, foresight, and self-control, all qualities that are not yet very well developed in children or teens. Recent findings from developmental neurobiology strongly support the idea of a *maturity gap* in adolescence, between well-developed reasoning skills but poor ability to use those skills, especially in social situations and in the "heat of the moment." The evidence also points to over-reactivity in the social-emotional reward system, with a concurrent increase in (often risky) reward-seeking behavior that the cognitive control system is not yet able to regulate effectively. The preference for immediate reward over delayed rewards (or consequences) is exactly contrary to the perspective necessary to promote good adherence. Yet this preference is absolutely normative in teens.

The second conclusion largely follows from the first (and is supported by a wealth of data): giving youth *independence* for illness management more often than not results in declining adherence and worse illness control. It also does not seem to accomplish the hoped-for-aim of better preparing youth for self-management, as overly independent youth appear to have worse disease knowledge than those with a more appropriate mix of independence and support.

Third, positive *parent involvement* not only helps prevent these declines, but can buffer against the detrimental effects of chronic stress that have derailed more than one youth, and that seem to hit children from impoverished families especially hard. Strengthening parent-child relationships may help buffer against the worst of these effects and help promote adherence in patients from impoverished backgrounds. Positive or authoritative parenting also moderates the risk and risk-taking behavior that characterize adolescence.

Fourth, the research literature is also clear that parenting can have negative effects on adherence when it is perceived as overly controlling, intrusive, or critical, and when parents and youth fall into a cycle of conflict around illness management. Helping parents support their children's *decision-making autonomy* is likely to be more effective in fostering development of self-care skills (with less risk for conflict) than prematurely pushing youth to become independent in their management.

Fifth, the disparities in adherence and overall health that currently plague minorities do not have to be as wide as they currently are. In much the way that a decline in adherence in adolescence often reflects a breakdown in family teamwork, problematic adherence among minorities often reflects the breakdown (or lack) of effective teamwork between families and their healthcare providers. While some of the difficulty in establishing family-provider teamwork may reflect implicit biases and distrust of the medical profession, perhaps the primary factor is problematic *communication*. Research has shown that healthcare providers often speak differently to their minority patients, asking less about their lives and quality of life, and using more biomedical language. Improving provider-patient communication can potentially go a long way in ameliorating disparities in adherence.

Sixth, the most effective interventions for addressing nonadherence tend to involve behavioral therapies, which is not surprising when one considers that adherence is first and foremost a behavior (or set of behaviors). However, interventions can be improved by including patient education and addressing psychosocial comorbidities such as depression. These interventions tend to be designed to be used by psychologists, or other professionals with expertise in behavioral health. The importance of having a psychologist on the multidisciplinary healthcare team is being increasingly recognized.

Seventh, nonadherence can become entrenched and difficult to manage once it has become a set pattern. Risk screening at diagnosis can help identify patients at-risk for problematic adherence, and thus provides the basis for preventive intervention. At the same time, nonadherence can occur at any point in the course of an illness, as the result of burnout, developmental changes, or situational changes in the life of the patient and the family. Thus, there is also a strong need for ongoing surveillance for adherence difficulties. As self-report often inflates actual adherence rates, more objective methods (e.g., electronic monitoring, daily diaries) can be used, but these can be costly or burdensome on families.

Eighth, adherence problems may be more efficiently addressed through triage models that allocate promotion and intervention resources based on assessed risk or need, such as Kazak's (2006) Pediatric Psychosocial Preventive Health Model (PPPHM). Most patients and families will have adequate coping and supports, and can be provided with universal educational materials and illness management tools to help promote adherence. A smaller subset will have risk factors for problematic adherence but no current clinical concerns. These patients and families could benefit from targeted interventions focused on ameliorating the indentified risk. Finally, a minority will present with clinically significant child or family dysfunction or very problematic adherence, requiring individualized treatment. Validated tools are available to help categorize level of risk/need.

Ninth, developing partnerships between patients, families, and providers may not be enough without also changing the *system* in which care is provided. The current healthcare system is overwhelmingly complex and too difficult for many families to navigate. For example, studies have shown that the majority of people are unable to complete insurance application forms without making mistakes. When patients are treated at large hospitals or medical centers, it can be difficult simply to know who to call to get questions answered, let alone reach the appropriate staff. Help with navigating systems is critical, especially for patients and families with lower health literacy.

Tenth, families often face more than one challenge or barrier when trying to manage a chronic illness. This is especially true of the most vulnerable families (Anderson 2012), who often face multiple risk factors simultaneously, including poverty, racial/ethnic minority status, mental illness and chronic disease among multiple family members, and substantial environmental and social stressors that can become "toxic." Interventions focused on only one facet of a multidimensional array of difficulties are unlikely to be very effective. Taking a systematic approach that integrates multi-level interventions has the potential to better help those families for whom nonadherence is not simply a one-dimensional problem.

In this volume we have argued that fostering healthcare partnerships around illness management has significant potential to improve adherence and children's health. Yet it has to be acknowledged that working together is not always easy. In fact, adherence may be so difficult in part because working together can be so difficult. Patients, providers, and parents each have their own views, their own goals, and often wish to go their own ways, and it can be quite challenging to bridge the gaps between them. Yet there will also be important areas of overlap—most obviously, in everyone's desire for the child to be healthy, and to have as near normal a life as can be achieved. Pediatricians and other primary care providers are well situated to help their patients and families find the areas of overlap. The greatest value of promoting teamwork around illness management may not even come from its impact on adherence, but from making chronic illness just a little bit less of a burden that a child has to carry around each day.

References

Anderson BJ. Who forgot? The challenges of family responsibility for adherence in vulnerable pediatric populations. Pediatrics. 2012;129(5):e1324–5.

Graves MM, Roberts MC, Rapoff M, Boyer A. The efficacy of adherence interventions for chronically ill children: a meta-analytic review. J Pediatr Psychol. 2010;35:368–82.

Kazak AE. Pediatric Psychosocial Preventative Health Model (PPPHM): research, practice and collaboration in pediatric family systems medicine. Fam Syst Health. 2006;24:381–95.

Kuehni CE, Frey U. Age-related differences in perceived asthma control in childhood: guidelines and reality. Eur Respir J. 2002;20:880–9.

Wysocki T. The ten keys to helping your child grow up with diabetes. Alexandria: American Diabetes Association; 1997.

Index

© Springer International Publishing Switzerland 2015
D. D. Schwartz, M. E. Axelrad, *Healthcare Partnerships for Pediatric Adherence,*
SpringerBriefs in Public Health, DOI 10.1007/978-3-319-13668-4

Printed in the United States
By Bookmasters